FAITH AND FURY

JYOTI YADAV is an award-winning journalist. Known for her fearless ground reporting at *ThePrint*, she has established herself as a long-form writer-reporter, capturing, over the past decade, social shifts that lurk unnoticed beneath 'breaking news' cycles. She is a chronicler of life in rural and small-town India at a time when journalism has shifted its focus to big cities and metropolitan urbanism.

Born and brought up in a village in Haryana, she fought her way out of the state's patriarchal setup to reach the National Capital, becoming the first person in her agrarian family to go to university and pursue postgraduate studies.

In 2020–21, she was one of the few journalists to cover the migrant exodus, the deadly second wave, and the pandemic's far-reaching impact on the hinterland in Bihar and Uttar Pradesh.

For her work, she has been awarded many national and international honours, including the prestigious Ramnath Goenka Award 2020, Journalist of the Year 2023 by the Indian Institute of Mass Communication, Young Journalist of the Year Award 2022 by the Thomson Foundation, the Statesman Award for Rural Reporting 2023, True Story Award 2024, the International Press Institute (IPI) Award 2022, and the UN Laadli Media Award for three consecutive years.

'Jyoti Yadav has the rare ability to capture the current churn in rural and small-town India. She brought this to her COVID coverage for *ThePrint*, travelling with migrant workers, exposing state capacity gaps in public healthcare, and diving into private pain and family distress. This book is an honest chronicle of the pandemic from the ground.'

—**Shekhar Gupta**, Editor-in-Chief, *ThePrint*

'This book is field journalism at its finest: telling compelling stories with a human touch about one of the most difficult periods in contemporary society. The COVID pandemic affected millions of lives, but beyond the statistics, it's the personal stories that matter. Jyoti Yadav's impactful journalism brings to life the agony and trauma of a disruption like no other.'

—**Rajdeep Sardesai**, senior journalist, *India Today*

'Jyoti Yadav has produced a remarkable record of India's pandemic years. It is perhaps for this reason that journalism is often referred to as the first draft of history. Through meticulous ground reporting across North India, Jyoti has documented the human cost of policy failures, the collapse of rural health infrastructure, and the resilience of our people. The book combines rigorous reporting with genuine empathy in the best traditions of long-form journalism, never letting tall claims or data obscure the faces and voices of ordinary Indians who lived through extraordinary tragedy.'

—**Prof. Manoj Kumar Jha**, MP (Rajya Sabha)

'Jyoti Yadav has written this book with extraordinary simplicity and clarity. Her reporting serves many purposes. *Faith and Fury* is a fascinating and valuable documentation of the COVID era. Yadav is a modern woman and a liberal writer with her roots in desi India, and the best part of the book is her emotional connection with the aam aadmi. She shares their pain and stories without trying to dominate the debate.'

—**Sheela Bhatt**, senior journalist

'This book is an immense reporting achievement. Battling frequent exhaustion, bouts of sickness, troll abuse, searing heat, abysmal sanitation, unreliable statistics and official resistance to truth-telling, Jyoti Yadav gives us a riveting chronicle of the unremitting tragedy that COVID was, especially in UP and Bihar, and the resilience that also sometimes accompanied it. Both urban and rural settings and the different rhythms of their healthcare are covered. Lucknow, Varanasi, Jaunpur, Patna, Darbhanga and Bodhgaya, among others, are sketched with keen observation and engaging writing. A must read.'

—**Ashutosh Varshney**, Sol Goldman Professor of International Studies and Political Science, Brown University, USA

'Jyoti Yadav's book is a stellar reminder of how ground reporting is a crucial pillar of democracy. Her travels to remote parts of India during the COVID-19 pandemic weave a complete picture of how the country's most vulnerable gasped for life. Her kind of shoe-leather journalism is so rare and inspiring. This book is a must read for anyone who wants to know how the lack of preparedness and a broken health and social infrastructure cost millions of Indian lives, and how we still have learnt so little since then. An important documentation that will shape Indian history.'

—**Neha Dixit**, senior journalist and author of *The Many Lives of Syeda X*

FAITH AND FURY

COVID DISPATCHES FROM INDIA'S HINTERLANDS

JYOTI YADAV

WESTLAND
NON·FICTION

WESTLAND
NON·FICTION

Published by Westland Non-Fiction, an imprint of Westland Books, a division of Nasadiya Technologies Private Limited, in 2026

No. 269/2B, First Floor, 'Irai Arul', Vimalraj Street, Nethaji Nagar, Alapakkam Main Road, Maduravoyal, Chennai 600095

ISBN: 9789371970983

10 9 8 7 6 5 4 3 2 1

Typeset by Jojy Philip

Printed at Parksons Graphics Pvt. Ltd

For

Imara and Rahul

Contents

Prologue

20 MARCH 2020

The ride from Mayur Vihar Metro Station to ITO was no longer like the one I had taken over the years. I don't recall which song was playing on my earphones that day, but I do remember scrolling through Twitter, pausing at tweets that seemed alarming.

The government kept telling us that Coronavirus wasn't a health emergency,[1] and we need not panic, and yet offices and corporations had already begun responding in quiet, decisive ways. Employees were beginning to work from home.

Over the past week, the number of passengers on the metro had been shrinking each day bit by bit. Before this time, empty seats used to be a rarity during the rush hour. The mad dash to grab seats was missing even in the ladies' coach. Nobody stood too close to you either, as in the past.

When I walked into the Express building, many offices on various floors had only guards at the gates; employees were working from home. In our newsroom, everyone had sky-blue surgical masks on their faces. A large bottle of sanitiser, tied to an iron pole, stood at the entrance. The biometric attendance system had been taped off. We were asked not to touch anything unnecessarily anymore.

The pantry, once buzzing with the chatter of reporters—hurriedly calling out to Basant Kumar the tea seller to come and serve tea before we stormed into the editorial room—had fallen silent. No more than four people could gather there at one time.

The desks in the hall were suddenly pushed apart, making close coworkers into distant neighbours. It gave a temporary relief for those of us who often fought for enough space around our desks. The new posters on the washroom walls reminded us to sanitise our hands more often.

That day, the 11 a.m. meeting wasn't held in the editorial room but was held outside it. Reporters remained seated at our desks, some stood with their notebooks, as our editor began asking for ideas. It honestly felt strange and surreal, as if it were part of some drill before a war or a sci-fi. That was the day it truly sank in. That, all of this was real. At 4:17 p.m. on 20 March 2020, an email flashed on my laptop screen. It was from my editor-in-chief, Shekhar Gupta. The email was marked to everyone at *ThePrint*.

> Dear all,
> We are now dealing with what could be the biggest story of our lives. We, the kinship of Indian journalism, will be tested as never before. Future generations of Indians will hold us to this. Let's recall that famous World War II poster: So where were you in the Great War, Grandpa/ma? It is that kind of moment for us. This is a deadly global pandemic.

A moment before this, I was on the phone with Satish (name changed to protect his identity), a fourth-grade contractual employee with the Ministry of Skill Development and Entrepreneurship (MSDE) in New Delhi. On 18 March, Satish was roaming on the third floor of Shram Shakti Bhawan, announcing that everyone should stay away from him because his mother had tested positive for COVID-19. The office of Union Skill Development Minister Mahendra Nath Pandey was located in the same building.

The news had spread like fire. Media WhatsApp groups were bombarded with messages from editors to follow up because this was one of the first cases of Coronavirus to have emerged from within the country, affecting an employee in a top ministry with no history of recent travel.

Until then, most reported cases had been linked to those who had travelled outside the country and brought the virus with them. Every reporter I knew was hot on the trail of this story, so I too called up the ministry's media contact, Garima Misra, who worked as government relations and lead communication advisor at the ministry, to confirm the lead. But she denied it. As more and more reporters pressed her for a confirmation, she decided to send out a press note that read, 'A contractual employee of the ministry has claimed that his mother has been detected with COVID-19. The concerned individual along with the others with whom he interacted have been asked to self-quarantine themselves at their residence. Their health will be closely monitored for further symptoms.

Further advice from the health ministry has been sought. The MSDE continues to follow the advisory of the Ministry of Health on precautionary measures to be taken for the purpose of social distancing, including usage of sanitisers and thermal temperature check.'[2]

Such was the panic that everyone in Shram Shakti Bhawan was recalling stories of meeting or shaking hands with Satish. Hundreds of employees who sat on the various floors were awaiting the next development with great anticipation. Every detail was decisive. Every piece of information would decide what the coming days in their lives would look like. As the day progressed, the uncertainty mounted. By evening, it turned out to be a rumour.

Everybody was looking for Satish; he had managed to shake the whole of Shram Shakti Bhawan. I managed to trace Satish through a source. 'Why did you spread such a rumour?' was my first question to him. He was silent for a moment, then answered, 'I wanted a leave. It looked like a good excuse.' I burst out laughing.

'I didn't anticipate this response, didn't think that the entire machinery would get after me. I never imagined this level of fear,' he pleaded innocence. But the damage had been done. He was sacked from his job. That day, on 20 March, India reported 234 positive cases of COVID-19.[3]

The deadly virus had already taken 10,000 lives worldwide by then and there were around 2.4 lakh active cases globally.[4]

Only four deaths had been reported so far; tragedy was yet to unfold in India.[5]

Meanwhile, in my professional career as a journalist until this juncture, I had covered crime against women, the 2019 Lok Sabha elections, the Jharkhand assembly elections, pop culture, policy and rural India. I was hungry for more assignments, and so my reporting editor, Renu Agal, had handed me three ministries to cover in January 2020. I had started mapping the lanes in the ministries of Women and Child Development, Skill India and Agriculture. I had barely gotten familiar with Vigyan Bhawan, PTI, Shram Shakti Bhawan, Krishi Bhawan and Shashtri Bhawan—the places where policies are drafted. I was just beginning to find out which gates to enter, which lifts were meant for outsiders, which clerk was friendly—the kinds of details seasoned beat reporters swear by, when the country was thrown into this unprecedented crisis. All my plans of cultivating more sources and getting exclusive policy stories were put on hold.

Around me, everyone spoke only about the deadly virus. All sorts of misinformation was being circulated on social media and WhatsApp. The air was thick with collective anxiety. The virus would soon take over the lives of millions of people. In certain areas, people were panic buying; ration shops were running out of essential supplies; there were long queues outside shopping marts.

Then, on 19 March 2020, Prime Minister Narendra Modi appeared on our screens.

He appealed to citizens to observe Janta Curfew between 7 a.m. and 9 p.m. on 22 March.

This got everyone excited and soon the curfew turned into a festival. Thalis and taalis were banged to show solidarity with health workers. Bunglows of district magistrates and superintendents of police in some parts of the country were lit with diyas, making it seem as though Diwali had arrived early that year, without the soft, fragrant breeze of October and November. Some celebrities and influencers even uploaded videos explaining the 'scientifically proven' benefits of the sound produced by clapping and ringing of bells—as a measure to kill Coronavirus.

On 24 March, the prime minister appeared on our screens once again, but this time to announce the extension of the curfew: 'From midnight today, listen carefully, from midnight today, the entire country will go into a complete lockdown. To save each citizen, you and your family, there will be a total ban on coming out of your homes. Every state, every union territory, every district, every small town, every village and every lane is being put under lockdown.'[6] 'Forget about leaving your homes for the next twenty-one days,' he further said.

The order became effective at 12.01 a.m., giving 1.3 billion Indians less than four hours to prepare for the lockdown.

International press called it the most severe step taken against the pandemic. 'The world's strictest lockdown,' wrote *The Guardian*.[7]

The joy of banging thalis did not last long. The prime minister's announcement triggered a massive migrant exodus—something that no one from my generation had ever witnessed. People were left on their own—unaware of the threat that the virus posed, unprepared for life in a lockdown and stranded in cities where they worked. The announcement of the lockdown did not allude to any plans for shelter or food. It did not take into account how people's jobs, and subsequently, lives, would be affected.

In no time, videos of chaotic scenes from bus stands in New Delhi, Gujarat, Rajasthan and Maharashtra went viral. The cities of India had started abandoning their watchmen, cooks, cleaners and daily wage workers.

Pictures of women carrying bundles on their heads and toddlers in their arms started emerging on social media. They were marching back to their villages.

On the other hand, media houses started laying off their employees—newspapers weren't being delivered anymore. There was also a change in the way newsrooms worked: the traditional editorial meeting was replaced with Zoom meetings, and discussions over story ideas took place on either WhatsApp or email. The lines between work and home blurred. There were times when the desk editor at *ThePrint* would call me to resolve (reply to playback or get quotes for the stories,) queries, and I would be doing the dishes. Amidst all this, a new reporting beat was created—the COVID beat.

India was about to face the worst health crisis since Independence, and no one knew how the situation was going to pan out. Every day, the nation awaited the crucial press briefings from the Union Health Ministry with bated breath.

Speaking on behalf of the ministry, Luv Aggarwal, an IIT graduate and IAS officer from Andhra Pradesh, had become India's face against the Coronavirus. He would brief the media about the availability of ICU beds, lockdown, testing, infection rates, active and recovered COVID-19 cases. He became a household name.

But what was missing in his briefings were the videos and images of migrants crying helplessly as they faced a brutal police crackdown. Even as they marched barefoot in the merciless summer heat, no one in the government was talking about them. Despite the fact that the videos and pictures of migrant workers were hard to ignore.

After filing an initial report from the Ghazipur border, I realised that I could understand their plight. But to truly be able to comprehend the scale of the exodus, I needed to be among the migrants. I sent a message to my editor, expressing my will to travel to Uttar Pradesh and Bihar to cover the migrant exodus. In April, the heartbreaking scenes of migrants—including pregnant women, toddlers and senior citizens—walking thousands of kilometres to reach their homes put India to great shame for having failed its poorest.

On the night of 6 May, I finally received the go-ahead from the managing editor at *ThePrint* to cover the migrant exodus. Most people advised me not to take the assignment.

'Jaan hai toh jahaan hai,' my friends and well-wishers said to me. Renu Agal, my immediate boss, called up and shared a few tips. 'Biscuits, water bottles, namkeen, masks and sanitizer, etc. You will need all these things as everything will be shut. No dhabas and no hotels will be open. Take hot water baths every morning and after returning from the assignment. Don't forget to wash your hair as the virus could be present in the hair too. Don't wear slippers, carry two pairs of shoes. Wash your clothes in Dettol and Surf because you will be visiting hospitals and migrants.'

I could not sleep that night. I had been briefed for a ten-day assignment, but I knew that it could easily take up to twenty or even thirty days. Once you are on the ground, you can't tell exactly when you will return. I called my colleague Bismee Taskin, who was to accompany me. My driver Manish was supposed to pick her up, then come to my place. Having been asked to leave for this mammoth of a story at such short notice, Bismee too was unprepared.

At 7 a.m. on the morning of 7 May 2025, we left for a reporting assignment that changed my worldview forever. In the next three weeks, we travelled across the Noida-Ghazipur border into Rampur, Bareilly, Sitapur, Hardoi, Lucknow, Sant Kabir Nagar and Gorakhpur districts in UP. Then we moved to Bihar, covering Gopalganj, Sitamarhi, Katihar, Bhagalpur, Purnea, Patna and Buxar districts.

As I traversed unfamiliar cities and towns, the rural-urban divide in India's health infrastructure revealed itself to me.

The idea of writing this book emerged after I returned from covering the migrant exodus. Minakshi Thakur, my editor, and I planned a book about the first COVID wave and the exodus, aiming to tell the story from a more human perspective rather than relying solely on statistics.

Then came the second wave, deadlier than the first, turning everything upside down. Once again, I found myself plunged into the COVID crisis in 2021. But a lot had changed in a year. If you ask me as a journalist, there was a striking difference between the two waves. In the first wave, we were the chroniclers of the catastrophe. But in 2021, many of us were losing our lives to the catastrophe. There is no concrete data available on the number of journalists who succumbed to the virus in India while doing their job, but it is estimated to be more than 500. Setting out to cover the pandemic yet again, I was at high risk of becoming a headline myself.

I recall a chief medical officer's warning from the Ghazipur district of Uttar Pradesh: 'In a war, you know who your enemy is, and you can anticipate their moves, but this virus is attacking from all sides. It is everywhere. Simply assume that everyone you meet out there is COVID-19 positive.'

Just as Shekhar had written in his email, 'we journalists have to defend justice and record history', *ThePrint*, a young newsroom in Indian media, was one of the few media organisations to send reporters to cover ground realities. And I was one of them.

Reporters are not supposed to get attached to a story; it biases them. But during the second wave, many journalists went way beyond the call of professional duty. We used our social media platforms to tweet SOS messages for hospital beds and oxygen cylinders; we spent nights writing stories and days coordinating with bureaucrats and hospitals. It was a twenty-four-hour shift. I once found myself standing in the middle of a crematorium in UP, counting dead bodies while tweeting for help for someone in need of urgent hospitalisation in Rajasthan. Even after tweeting for dozens of patients, at the end of the day, guilt would descend on me for not having been able to respond to all the distress calls. The emotional exhaustion was too great.

I have been working on this book for the last few years, trying to document the catastrophe faithfully and in a comprehensive manner. A book on COVID would be incomplete without examining rural and small-town India. So I spent a lot of time after 2021 revisiting the same places again and again, observing the changes—or lack thereof—in health infrastructure, human development indices, grassroots politics and the states' preparedness for crisis management in the aftermath of pandemic.

My journey began as a cub reporter with an insider's view of the rural world. Over time, I realised that understanding a diverse country like India could take a lifetime, and even then, one might still feel inadequate in their comprehension. The sheer size and diversity of India mean that a statement true for a group of 10,000 people might be completely untrue for another group of the same size. India is so full of paradoxes. In a true sense, it's a work in progress.

Both the COVID years—2020 and 2021—have left us with many questions. The pandemic shattered families across generations. It wiped out entire families and left millions grasping at straws haunted by regrets. 'Could we have bought that one oxygen cylinder, scraped together a few extra thousand rupees, and saved Papa?' Somewhere in a tier-two city, a son wrestles with this thought every night.

'What if I had begged one more time for a hospital bed—would my wife still be by my side today?' A father, now raising his children alone, carries inside him this question like a wound that never heals.

'We were orphaned within a matter of days, and life changed forever.' In a quiet village in Bihar, three children—COVID orphans—will someday tell their children, perhaps their grandchildren too, the story of those years.

Social media algorithms may have caused fatigue with regard to the word COVID. It may no longer be a keyword that gets the news industry a wide readership. In fact, there is a tendency to either skip or gloss over the news that mentions COVID-19. In newsrooms, a line is often tossed around that COVID has been 'written to death.'

This is true to some extent, but outside the realm of the Internet, in the real world, the COVID years haven't yet been forgotten. 2020 and 2021 mark a milestone in the life of an entire nation as well as the world. You meet any individual, and they will have a COVID story to tell. Some will be inspiring, while others will be harrowing. Just as Zora Neale Hurston, a pioneering Black anthropologist, writer and folklorist, spoke of the passage of time in her 1937 novel, *Their Eyes Were Watching God*: 'There are years that ask questions and years that answer.'

In May 2025, the Office of the Registrar General & Census Commissioner of India (ORGI) lifted the veil on the deaths in 2021—and suddenly, we were back to the questions of the COVID years.

The latest data revealed that India recorded 10.22 million registered deaths in 2021—a 25.9 per cent increase from the 8.12 million deaths in 2020. A staggering rise, 1.97 million additional deaths in just one year.

In those two years, there were no natural disasters or wars that would explain mortality at such scale. These numbers actually reveal an unseen, unaccounted for, toll taken by the virus.

Each year uncovers something about the COVID era. With each new revelation, we make a little more sense of what we went through collectively, where we failed, and where we succeeded. The search for answers continues.

This book—five years in the making—is a part of that search. The current news cycle may be done with COVID, but those years will not be forgotten. They will survive through the indelible scars on the families affected, and the data collated through ground reporting.

As for me, I wanted to record the faces, the stories, the goodbyes that have stayed with me from my travels during the time of COVID. This is an attempt to retrieve them from statistical records and make them count as lives that mattered.

1

A Long Way from Home

Manish Upadhyay, Bismee and I packed our suitcases and started in an Innova in the early hours of 6 May. We could only arrange a few bottles of sanitiser for the COVID kit that we were supposed to carry. There was a shortage of N-95 masks and PPE kits, even for the medical frontline workers, so we wore surgical masks.

In no time, we were on the highway. The lanes in Mayur Vihar and Noida were silent. There was barely any movement of vehicles. The shutters were down. The vegetable vendors, joggers, milkmen or even the usual morning crowd that we were used to seeing see while leaving for assignments in the early hours, were missing.

We did see a few cars but these were allowed on the road because they had been marked with 'essential service' stickers. Manish had brought a printout to stick to the front of the car. It said—'PRESS' in huge white and red letters.

We left Ghaziabad behind and moved further into UP. There was a police crackdown on the migrants who were marching home with their cycles and bundles of essentials. At many checkpoints, these migrants were being stopped by cops, put in vehicles and dropped off in quarantine centres miles away.

Many migrants had started taking different, and longer, routes by getting off the highway in order to avoid the initial police checkpoints established by the state for screening. But when we drove further into the rural belts, we saw the migrants returning to the highway. After walking longer routes, they ultimately had to return to the highway to stay on course. While the highway offered some relief, it also intensified their hardships, exposing them to the brutal force of the state. The vibrant highway culture of dhabas and tea stalls was no longer visible. The big restaurants had their staffers but they could not function either.

Our first stop was Rampur, about 200 kilometres from Delhi. Rampur is a northwestern rural district with a population of 23.36 lakh. It is known for its rich heritage and history. Its Raza Library, founded by the first nawab of Rampur, Nawab Faizullah Khan, in the eighteenth century, is considered an important centre for Indo-Islamic studies in South Asia.

But in the present-day, communally charged times, Rampur's identity has been reduced to that of a Muslim-dominated constituency, an idea on which political parties want to capitalise.

When we started our journey, India had been under lockdown for almost forty days. Now, states like UP and Bihar had started working on plans to help migrants return to their homes. But even after the aid of Shramik trains by the central government, it was common to see migrants trudging along highways, some walking and some others cycling.

The harvest season was due to begin soon, and farmers were getting anxious about their crops. Some of them started to move into their fields, while some awaited the district administration's guidelines.

Before entering Rampur, we had briefly stopped at a bus depot near Amroha on National Highway 24, which connects Lucknow to Delhi). Migrants were waiting there for state buses to ferry them home. Their bicycles had been abandoned on the sides of the road. When we spoke, they were caught in a dilemma—over whether to abandon their 'saathi' or not. Some made a difficult choice, but others sat on the roofs of buses clutching their cycles close to their hearts.

Every migrant had a story and each story was heartbreaking. As a reporter, picking one story over the others was difficult for me. But we had to find the ones that could resonate with millions, impacting thereby the policies that would be framed for them.

RAMPUR

We reached Rampur by the evening of 6 May. The district administration was busy implementing lockdown guidelines. Accessing the officials was challenging as most of them were hectically carrying out the multiple orders landing in their offices now and then from the state government.

We decided to visit the outer part of the town, venturing into a cluster of three villages—Agapur, Ajitpur and Mansurpur—located at a distance of just two kilometres from the Rampur railway station.[1]

The lockdown had turned the otherwise bustling lanes of these villages into a zone of distress and disappointment. Most elderly people sat idle on the verandas of their homes. Schools were shut and children spent long humid days of summer at home. The online learning system hadn't been rolled out yet in villages as in the urban parts of the country. (The online system of teaching was still being developed, and only the privileged sections of society were able to continue their education through their computers and phones. A significant gap in smart phone ownership among the masses meant that many children were left behind. It was only months later that NGOs and private groups began to realise that the pandemic had severely impacted the education of underprivileged children.)

Children either peeked outside from gates or played indoors. Some men and children, however, sat outside the shuttered shops. But there wasn't much to do. Their lives had come to a halt.

The first story that we decided to dispatch was about how an Indian village was collectively coping with the lockdown and its fallouts. We parked our car in a lane in Mansurpur. We got down with our lapel mics in place and a One-plus mobile to record interviews and started knocking on a few doors. It was the month of Ramzan. We met a watermelon seller who was roaming across the streets. He told us that this was a difficult time, especially for poor families like his that lived hand to mouth.

Nanni, a woman in her late forties, wearing an orange dupatta and off-white salwar-kameez, was peeping out from a nearby home. She saw us ringing her neighbour's bell. She seemed eager to start a conversation about her livelihood: selling buffalo milk. Nanni owned two buffaloes and two calves. When we asked her what had changed in the last forty days, she said that those who used to buy two litres of milk had cut down their milk intake to a litre or one and a half.

In another lane, we stopped by a grocery store run by Ameer Ahmed. He had been running it for the past twelve years. Logon ke paas kaam toh raha nahi. Jiski udhari 5,000 rupaye ki thi, ab wo badhkar zyada ho gayi hai,' he said. People are out of work. If someone had a loan of 5,000 rupees on their head earlier, it has increased considerably.

As we talked to more people, we found out that these three villages, much like the rest of rural India, had been hit hard by the lockdown. Farmers too had incurred losses.

We also met Rustom Hussain, a farmer, who said that he had to sell his harvest at a throwaway price. 'We have no other option but to bear the losses. The government had promised that it would facilitate the sale of wheat at the MSP (Minimum Support Price) of Rs 1,925 per quintal, but nothing like that has happened in all this while. We have been forced to sell the crop to locals at Rs 1,720 per quintal,' he said. Harvesting was already delayed by the unavailability of labour and combine harvesters due to the lockdown. Many farmers who had decided to store their harvest and fetch good prices later were getting anxious. Overall, the situation in villages was getting more and more distressing and confusing by the day.

We left the villages at dusk and started looking for accommodation. All the hotels on the national highway along Rampur were shut.

I called up my colleague Praveen Jain, the national photo editor at *ThePrint*. He, one of my other colleagues Simrin and their driver Anil had tested positive in the last week of April and were quarantined in Vadodara, Gujarat. They had been on the road since 11 April, covering Jaipur, Ajmer, Kota, Udaipur and Ahmedabad along the way. Their last stop was Vadodara where they had caught the virus.

Praveen connected me to one of the hotel owners he knew from his previous assignments near Rampur. We reached the hotel, and while it was shut, the owner came to meet us outside the gate. He said he was entirely helpless and could not let us stay due to the strictness of the police's decree. 'But you are always welcome to visit us when things go back to being normal.' He promised to be a good host in the future.

Left with no option but to leave, we began driving towards the next district, Bareilly, around seventy kilometres away. We had gone only a few kilometres on NH 24 when we spotted some people hiding behind trees in the fields.

When they saw us approaching, they ran away. Only when we assured a local farmer, who had come to offer food and water to them, that we were neither police nor administration, did he summon them back. They were hiding from the police. The farmer called out to them, 'Arey, media waale hain. Tumhari samasya sunne aaye hain.' They are from the media. They only want to highlight your plight. So they sat down with us and opened up.

'If we get caught, the police send us back to quarantine centres and delay our journey.' One of the eight migrant workers explained that they were taking a short break as they had been on their feet for eight days at a stretch, walking from Haryana to their native villages in Gorakhpur district.

Arvind, a lean, acutely tanned man in his late thirties, said, 'I haven't eaten a morsel of roti since I started walking.'

'I had carried some belongings but had to get rid of them midway as I couldn't drag the load,' Dharmraj said.

Ramu, the third migrant, spoke about the brutality and apathy of the state, 'Some of us have already spent a few days in quarantine centres. If another district's police nabs us now, our two-three-day journey will get extended by six more days.

Before he could finish his sentence, he broke down. 'I just want to see my children.'

By the time the migrants finished telling their stories, the local farmer had become agitated about the government not having made any arrangements for the poor workers.

'Every day we see 20,000 to 25,000 people crossing this highway. We can't bear to watch their suffering. So whatever little we can do, like providing food and water, we are doing.'

On this note, we ended our assignment for the day. The state may not have spared a thought for the migrants, but the villages they crossed were offering them shelter, food and the comforting words, 'they were not alone'.[2]

BAREILLY

We had left for Bareilly in the hope of finding accommodation, but ended up chasing a very crucial story: the Shramik trains.

On our way to the district headquarters, we found buses and trucks filled with people. They had walked thousands of kilometres; they were tired, helpless and lonely. Buses and trucks were parked outside petrol pumps as they navigated the guidelines that each district administration had enforced.

It was at dawn that we got into one of the buses to talk to those who could afford the fare to return home. To our surprise, they had endured the same hardship and suffering as those who were penniless. They were paying as much as 5,000 rupees per seat. Even for a ride on a truck loaded with concrete, a migrant worker had paid a 1,000 rupees.

We reached the town late in the evening. We seemed to have lost our bearings. This place was unfamiliar to all of us. It was Bismee's first on-ground assignment outside Delhi. I had already spent a year on the road, but I had never been to Bareilly. So, there weren't many sources we could rely on.

Still without a place to stay (and periodically calling our friends in Delhi for help), we made our way to the railway station. A Shramik Express was due to arrive with more than a 1,000 migrants from Punjab's Ludhiana. Policemen, railway officials and district officials were all set to welcome the migrants with packets of food and water. While the policemen wore face shields and other officials had gloves on, the migrants had their white gamchhas wrapped around their faces as makeshift masks.

After an eleven-hour train journey without any halts, or food or water, when they got down at Bareilly Junction, there was temporary relief on the tired and restless faces of the migrants. Healthcare workers screened the migrants while sanitation workers sprayed disinfectants around the platform.

Forty-three buses had been arranged to drop people off at their respective districts and blocks. When a wave of migrants rushed to the buses, the police, anticipating chaos, were on the alert. They started announcing the number plates of the buses and the places they would head to.

As Bismee and I waited at a distance, we spotted twenty-eight–year–old Nooni Ram anxiously looking for the bus that would take him to Aonla town, a tehsil in Bareilly district, about sixty kilometres away.

But his journey wouldn't end in Aonla. He, his wife and their child would travel a further eighteen kilometres to reach Hardaspur, their village.

'If we don't get conveyance, we will have to walk eighteen kilometres to get home,' Nooni Ram said as he showed us a message on his phone.

'We got a message from the office of district magistrate, Ludhiana at 10 o' clock in the night that the train for Bareilly will start at three in the morning. We got only five hours to pack and reach the station. How are we supposed to prepare for anything at such short notice?' he asked.

The message also said that they would be allowed to board the train only if they cleared the COVID test screening.

'Bring your own food and water. Punjab government wishes you a safe journey,' that's how the message ended. A 1,000 migrant families didn't catch a wink that night. They had left in whatever condition they were; some couldn't even pack their bags, so they threw their things in buckets and carried them. The five-hour notice was nowhere near enough for people who lived far away from the railway station.

Nooni Ram's wife fed her two-and-a-half–year–old from the food packet the couple had received upon their arrival, the child sitting between them as the bus headed home. We never found out if the family of three found a ride home or walked the last eighteen kilometres to their home in the dead of night.

The first Shramik train was flagged off on 1 May, the International Labour Day. In the days that followed, Shramik trains would have brought Nooni Ram and thousands like him to the Bareilly station.

But the humiliation that migrants like Nooni Ram were subjected to in the days that followed was appalling. They were already out of jobs. They had limited ration on their plates and mere pennies in their pockets. Their plight was made worse by the haggling between the states and the Centre. The Centre got caught up in political tussles in the states where opposing parties were in power, leading to a lack of coordination between them. One glaring example of this was the mismanagement of Shramik trains, including the poor food and travel arrangements for migrants.

Like every other government aid, this too was politicised. On 2 May, the railway ministry notified the state governments that they were to collect the ticket fare from migrants and hand the amount over to the railways.[3]

This move triggered a social media storm. The netizens ran a campaign on how the railways had 151 crore rupees to donate to the Prime Minister's Citizen Assistance and Relief in Emergency Situations Fund (PM CARES Fund) but not enough to run these special trains.[4]

The opposition vehemently criticised the decision. The Congress's then interim president Sonia Gandhi even announced that her party would foot the ticket fares.[5] The government then said that the cost would be borne by the Centre and the states at a 85 per cent: 15 per cent split.[6]

At this stage in the lockdown and COVID crisis, local administrations across Indian states were not just setting up quarantine centres, marking containment zones, managing Shramik trains that arrived in their districts, screening the lakhs of the migrants and arranging food for them, providing shelter to the homeless, creating employment, compiling a real time database, but also attending to thousands of SOS calls, regulating permissions for emergency travel, etc.

The Centre's role should have been that of an advisor, a facilitator laying down SOPs for the states so that each state could fight its battles in a more organised way. For example, district magistrates in several districts of Bihar had, two weeks before the national lockdown, imposed Section 144 to disperse large gatherings and curb the spread of the virus. However, the Centre was wary of spreading unnecessary panic since the severity of fatalities and the virus's controllability remained uncertain until then.

The orders were rolled back when the health ministry said that Coronavirus wasn't a medical emergency.

If the states had been afforded some autonomy in crisis management, the state and district decisions would have been far less harsh than a complete, nationwide lockdown, which froze all activity in the country. The Centre tried to take charge but ended up creating chaos and confusion. The BJP's national spokesperson, Sambit Patra, lashed out at Rahul Gandhi: 'The Railways has subsidised 85% and the state governments should pay 15%.'[7]

But in reality, the central government didn't pay 85 per cent of the fare, it admitted in the Supreme Court on 28 May during a virtual hearing on a PIL about the hardships faced by migrants stranded in different states amidst the lockdown. They clarified that the cost was borne by the states.[8]

Punjab, like several other states, had created an online portal to help migrant workers register themselves. 6.44 lakh migrants registered.[9] The government had sanctioned a budget of 35 crores in the first phase to send stranded migrants back to their home states. Hence this chatter over most of the cost being borne by the Railways remained a hot political debate until K.B.S. Sidhu, Punjab Special Chief Secretary, Revenue, hit back.[10]

The Punjab government also ordered all the deputy commissioners in the state to provide food, snacks and water to the migrants.[11] However, Nooni Ram and his fellow passengers did not receive food or water.

It was a hectic day for us. We had reported two stories: one, of the marching migrants being randomly nabbed by the police and thrown into quarantine centres; and two, the facts about Shramik trains. It was yet again time to find lodgings. Another colleague of mine, helped us find a hotel that arranged some home-cooked food for Manish, Bismee and me. The hotel rooms had been shut for more than a month and they smelt bad. Most of the staff had left so the place was running with just two or three men, but we couldn't complain. We ate our dinner and sat down to type our stories and send the video footage to our colleagues in Delhi. Both the stories drew overwhelming attention and trolling. Our headline said thousands of migrants weren't given food and water. It didn't go down well with lots of people on online platforms. Comments such as, 'Now they want VIP treatment too. Are train tickets not enough?' started flooding our social media handles.

In September 2020, when three Members of Parliament—Kani K. Navaskani, Suresh Narayan Dhanorkar and Adoor Prakash—asked the Ministry of Labour and Employment exactly how many migrants had died during the lockdown, the ministry replied that there was no data) available to ascertain that.[12]

A week later, replying to Trinamool Congress MP Derek O'Brien's question in the Rajya Sabha about migrant casualties on Shramik trains, the then minister for railways, Piyush Goyal said that ninety-seven migrants had died on Shramik trains.[13] Out of those, the state police had sent eighty-seven bodies for postmortem. The centre had obtained fifty-one postmortem reports from the states which indicated that the reasons for the deaths varied from cardiac arrest, heart disease, brain hemorrhage to pre-existing chronic diseases like chronic lung disease, chronic liver disease, and so on.

MGNREGA

The next morning, on 7th May, we discussed a few story ideas. We didn't know anyone in the city. Incidentally, a banker posted in Bareilly who had been following my ground reports for a long time messaged me on Facebook offering assistance and food.

Relieved, we landed up at his home around 11 a.m. and ate brunch. He then offered to accompany us to some of the nearby villages he was familiar with.

The first village we went to was called Ghunsa. It was on the outskirts of Bareilly. Every village we passed through had the same story: many migrants had walked home in the months of March and April; there were some who were taking buses and trains home now; and many were still stranded in other states. The ones who were home described the great hardships they had faced along the way. On reaching, they had been sheltered in government schools serving as quarantine centres for two weeks before being sent home.

And now, they needed work.

We spent the entire day going from village to village, after which we set up a meeting with Bareilly's chief development officer (CDO), Chandra Mohan. A CDO, second only to the district magistrate, oversees the execution of poverty alleviation, infrastructure, education, health and development schemes of the state and the central government. Chandra Mohan. a 2016 batch IAS officer, was working on rolling out a few schemes for the benefit of the migrants who had returned. We met him in his office the next afternoon.

He spoke about MGNREGA (Mahatma Gandhi National Rural Employment Guarantee Act) becoming a lifeline for the migrants who had returned.

Districts across India had started enrolling returned migrants under MGNREGA. Bareilly, at this time, employed about 47,000 workers under MGNREGA, including the migrants. The scheme covered 879 villages in the district.

MGNREGA is an employment guarantee scheme that was launched in 200 districts in February 2006, and is now considered to be the largest employment programme in the world. The act mandates a minimum of a hundred days of guaranteed wage employment in a financial year to at least one member of every rural household with adults who volunteer to perform unskilled manual work. MGNREGA was repealed and replaced by the VB-GRAMG Bill (Viksit Bharat—Guarantee for Rozgar and Ajeevika Mission (Gramin) Bill) in December 2025 by the Modi government.

A report published by Azim Premji University in October 2022 states that MGNREGA became a safety net despite its shortcomings.[14]

'The study found that MGNREGA made a marked difference during the pandemic, protecting the most vulnerable households from significant loss of income. Increased earnings from MGNREGA were able to compensate for somewhere between 20% to 80% of income loss depending on the block.'[15]

In the case of Bareilly, Chandra Mohan said that following the unprecedented influx of migrants, the employment rate under MGNREGA went up five times. He also shared the names of a few villages where MGNREGA activities were ongoing, and connected us with a few block-level officials who would provide further insights into the kind of labour being performed by workers availing the MGNREGA.

We had somehow managed to secure N-95 masks in Bareilly.

Many in the journalistic fraternity were questioning the decision to send reporters from Delhi to other parts of the country and putting their lives at risk. But the risk had to be taken because the story wasn't in Delhi, but on the ground. Nobody wanted to get infected and quarantined in a place far away from home. I panicked more than my colleagues.

I still have photos in my phone gallery where I am seen sanitising my phone for the millionth time. Every time I returned to the car, I would wipe my glasses, phone and even slippers, with sanitiser. Bismee and Manish were in better spirits; they would often crack jokes to diffuse my anxiety.

We were meeting migrants in buses, trucks and on the road. Anyone could be asymptomatic and pass on the virus to others. Imagine the social media trolling we would be subjected to if we were found infected at any point during our assignment.

After finishing the interview with CDO Chandra Mohan, we were on our way. We reached a village called Bilpur in Faridpur Tehsil, located at the border of Shahjahanpur and Bareilly districts.

The block officials with whom the CDO had connected us were present on the site. A Savlon handwash dispenser and sanitiser were neatly kept next to a blue bucket filled with water.

Here, about 110 migrant workers were employed to build a chak road. It was basically a kucha road that was being dug manually by the workers. It would connect Bilpur to the neighbouring village, Khajuri. The work on this road had started seven days ago and it was about to be completed. Each worker would get a daily wage of 202 rupees.

'This chak road will prevent rainwater from flooding the farms, enable people to access tractors for ploughing and make going from one village to the other easy,' the Gram Pradhan, Jitendra Verma, explained to us.

We spent over two hours at the site.

'Of the 110 workers employed here, thirty-five migrant workers returned on foot from the cities. They have no source of income in the village,' said the Gram Pradhan.

Majority of the migrants were either landless or owned a small piece of land that was not sufficient to meet the needs of their families. People from this village had gone to Delhi and Mumbai in search of work. They were among the first to leave the cities in the last week of March and arrived in their villages in early April. By May, they were looking for work to feed their families.

When we met twenty-five–year–old Dinesh Singh, he was digging soil. In Delhi, he had worked at a sweet shop in Badarpur. The day the PM announced the lockdown, he decided to leave for home.

'I wasn't feeling well in Delhi, and was really scared of getting infected with COVID-19. The food in the sweet shop had started decaying ... There wasn't anything left to hang on to there. Survival became really tough.' Singh said he had walked from Badarpur to Ghaziabad, where he came across a Tata 407 transporting milk. The driver was kind enough to give him and a few other migrants a lift. In Rampur, Dinesh and the lot were stopped by cops who took their temperature, screened them for symptoms and quarantined them for two weeks. It had been weeks since the police brought him to his village after his quarantine. The sole bread earner of his family, he earned 8,500 rupees a month in Delhi. Now, he had turned to MGNREGA.

Ved Prakash, another migrant at the same site, used to work as a railway labourer in Old Delhi, earning 350 rupees a day. He had left on 27 March, walked for ten straight days and reached Bilpur. 'I couldn't find any food or water for two-three days, but I didn't stop,' he recalled. Now, for Ved Prakash and his father this was their fifth day of digging the chak road.

LUCKNOW

On 8 May, we started on the Lucknow-Hardoi-Shahjahanpur highway to reach our next stop, Lucknow. But as we were crossing Hardoi, we saw groups of people stranded on the roadside. They had taken shelter under trees. They were waiting for trucks, requesting truck drivers to help them reach their villages, or at least some of the way, but no one helped.

There were 1,188 of them when they arrived in the first Shramik train from Punjab's Mohali to UP's Hardoi on the night of 7 May. The district administration provided 1 kg potato and ration kits of 10 kg, which contained salt, flour and rice—which only made for extra burden on the remaining part of the migrants' journey. Along with their own luggage, they dragged the ration kits too with their tired hands.

They were taken to an empty government building to spend the night, and in the morning when they lost patience, the ground officials told them to either wait or find their own conveyance to go home.

This broke Sunaina's spirit. 'Looks like our distress won't ever end. Had they told us before, we would have tried to arrange something. Now what do we do with this scorching sun and our children? Our home (Bhagauli) is thirty-five kilometres away from here.' Sunaina worked at a dhaga (thread) mill in Mohali, Punjab.

Amit Kumar, who worked at the same dhaga mill, was sitting under a tree with seven members of his family, out of which four were children, including one infant and one toddler. Amit had made a few calls to Bhagauli a few hours ago and one of his relatives was now pulling up in a mini-truck. People watched eagerly as Amit and his family climbed into the truck and departed for home.

The others waiting by the roadside were so worn-out, they struggled to articulate their frustration.

'Don't know how to go home. We have been moving from one place to another for days, now we are just exhausted,' said Arun, a migrant worker from Sandana in Sitapur district, around thirty kilometres from Hardoi.

This report was published two days later with the headline 'Migrants Are Told to Find Their Own Way Home'.[16]

The additional district magistrate of Hardoi rebutted our report, saying it was 'misleading and based on twisted facts'.

We published not only the district administration's reply but also a rejoinder along with the migrants' video testimonies as proof. The district magistrate didn't respond to it. We remained focused on covering the crisis. Rebuttals are a part of reporting.

We entered Lucknow on the evening of 8 May. True to its fame, Lucknow stood out as the city of nawabs, with its old charm intact even in the midst of brand new infrastructure.

The hotels were all closed. 'But I am on it. I am trying to get you in somewhere,' Sangeeta Malhotra, manager in the admin at *ThePrint*, assured us over a phone call.

This was our third day of reporting and we had filed three text reports, three video stories and two photo galleries. I was also filing stories in Hindi. We were extremely hungry, sleep-deprived and dehydrated. Sangeeta managed to find a hotel in Gomti Nagar, but it had no staff.

We could not be seen entering through the main gate, so we scaled the back gate. It was almost 8 p.m. and there was no tea, food or even snacks. We hadn't had a meal all day. I called my colleague Praveen again. He was COVID positive but recovering well. He graciously connected us with his friend who was an SHO in one of Lucknow's police stations.

Soon, a policeman arrived on a bike with a parcel containing biscuits and muffins—barely enough for three. While Bismee and I filed our stories, Manish went into the city to find sustenance and returned with groceries. There was a stove in the basement that used to be a kitchen. Manish and the person who had opened the hotel for us cooked dal and rice. We were so grateful for the meal. We saved the biscuits and muffins for the road.

The next morning, we thought not just about the stories we would cover but also about how we could arrange food. A friend from Twitter (now X), Arvind Shukla, who at the time worked with *Gaon Connection* (India's first rural newspaper), lived in Lucknow with his wife Sadhana and two children. During the first wave, people were apprehensive about letting outsiders into their homes. The virus was mysterious and unpredictable; elders and children were especially at risk.

Arvind said that he avoided long, far-off assignments, choosing instead to work closer to home. 'You could bring the virus home, and I worry for my children,' he admitted his concerns over the phone call. This fear kept his doors closed to us at first.

But something changed after our second call.

Arvind and Sadhana went out of their way to help us. There was a rare kind of empathy in that gesture, the kind that requires you to put others before yourself.

We met for lunch. As we prepared to head off on our journey, Sadhana gave us a parcel—pooris, lovingly packed for the road ahead. Arvind walks his own path now as an independent journalist, establishing *News Potli*—a rural journalism portal like no other. It is raw, unfiltered and straight from the heart.

Another person whom I was connected with on Facebook, Vaibhav Maheshwari, offered to help us. When we reached his house, we were served tea outside. Then he handed over a few gamchhas and a packed meal that would last us two days. We bid them goodbye and left for Sitapur.

Sitapur is about eighty-eight kilometres away from Lucknow. On our way there, we saw three men pulling a thela on the highway. They were headed to their village, Haripur, with Kandahi, a thirty-six–year–old man, lying still on the thela, wrapped in a blue blanket.

Kandahi had gone to Lucknow twenty years ago to look for work, and he had found it at Sanjay Bhatta, a brick kiln. He had worked day and night since he was sixteen, until he fell sick on 5 May 2020.

'The brick kiln people brought him to the village in a pick-up truck. They said he had slept on a boulder and was coughing all night,' his uncle, Chhote lal, told us.

Kandahi's parents had died long ago; Chhote Lal was all he had. He took Kandahi to the district hospital the next day where he was diagnosed with bronchitis, a respiratory disease common among brick kiln workers. But within two days, Chhote Lal had decided to take him back to the village.

'He doesn't have any savings. Twenty years of work and there is not a single paisa in his pocket. There wasn't much the hospital was doing. He has become terribly sick and is unable to even move on his own.' Chhote Lal then tried to arrange an ambulance but it cost a 1,000 rupees.

'My village isn't that far, but due to the lockdown, prices have shot up,' he remarked. So, sixteen-year-old Sandeep and another man known to Chhote Lal borrowed a thela from a neighbour to transport Kandahi home from the district hospital.

We wanted to publish this story, but what would it be about? A person who worked in a brick kiln for twenty years and didn't have any savings to get treatment in a hospital? Or an uncle, a labourer himself, who couldn't afford an ambulance for a 1,000 rupees? Or Sandeep, who had dropped out of school to do manual labour? Or about the apathy of the kiln owner who had abandoned a worker during a crisis?

We never filed the story, but today when I think of it, I feel it should have been about a brick kiln labourer and his abandonment.

SITAPUR

Arvind Shukla had connected us with a reporter in Sitapur, whom we met before proceeding to the district headquarters. Sangeeta had exhausted her contacts, and she couldn't find us a hotel. Someone I knew in Lucknow came to the rescue. He knew someone who ran a banquet hall in Sitapur.

The hall had been shut since March. The staff were all from Uttarakhand—stuck here in the pandemic.

We were going to report from a tehsil called Biswan in northeastern UP the next day. We had identified two villages in Biswan tehsil—Durga Purwa and Nai Basti—separated by three rivers—Sharda, Ghagra and Saryu. Both were ninety kilometres away from the mainland district of Sitapur.

On 10 May, we started early in the morning. Ordinarily, it would have taken much longer to get there, but due to the lockdown, for miles we were the only ones on the road. This wasn't the route the migrants walked. On the other highways, all one saw was a sea of them.

In less than two hours, we were in Durga Purwa. This was a remote village. When we asked for directions to reach the village head, a few villagers volunteered to take us there. As we followed them into narrow lanes, many villagers started gathering around the car. They were curious to see three strangers. They weren't sure if we were journalists as we weren't carrying large cameras or travelling in an OB van. Although the car had 'PRESS' emblazoned on it, few could read or even notice it.

It was in fact very strange to not find a bunch of reporters seeking shelter in the same hotels that we secretly sneaked into, or at the bus depots where we shot our pieces to camera (PTCs), or at the railway stations we rushed to in order to collect bytes of migrants arriving in Shramik trains or even at the collectorates where we tried to meet district officials.

This was also the phase when text reports were filed on phone calls, interviews were recorded through zoom calls and photographs were sourced from locals.

Indian journalists have always braved storms and reported from epicentres, be it elections, protests, murders, rallies or humanitarian disasters.

In every crisis, you will find them in the midst of the chaos, dozens of reporters standing before cameras gripping their mics.

But the COVID crisis was exceptionally different.

This time, the cameras hesitated to cross borders. Delhi, Mumbai, Thane, Surat, Bhopal—the usual hotspots of reportage remained well covered. But when it came to following the migrants back home, the screens remained eerily silent.

A large part of the media's focus stayed on interstate borders, checkpoints and containment zones in the cities. Few crossed into the heart of rural India in those crucial early months. Especially between 15 April and 15 May.

It wasn't until the end of May and early June, when the chaos settled a little, that alternate media houses began piecing together fragments of the untold stories.

There were many explanations for this. One of them was the sheer challenge of travel. With no flights, no trains and not even buses, movement was brutally restricted. If you had the energy to cover overnight distances spanning hundreds of kilometres daily—moving from one city to another—you could report. Ground reporting is essentially about traveling, and when the means to reach the story gets restricted, it becomes challenging.

The travel itself came with many risks. Food was scarce. Not all cab drivers were willing to take passengers. The fear of fatality was very real. This deterred even the most seasoned reporters of this country.

Then, there was this—those who had the means to travel didn't have the courage or conviction to do so.

Early on in our assignment, a senior reporter from a major news channel had called me to ask how we were able to cross the checkpoints in every district, where we stayed, where we ate and lastly, how to dodge the virus while doing so.

Some others reached out too, saying *ThePrint*'s coverage had sparked something within them and given them the impetus to hit the road.

When the second wave struck, many journalists weighed their choices carefully, calculating when it was safest to set out.

Some ventured out only after vaccination, others after recovering from COVID, hoping immunity would shield them from falling sick in the thick of the crisis. And for many, the turning point came when the number of cases finally began to decline.

In the thick of it all, I found myself in a rare position—alongside my colleagues—bearing witness to one of the gravest countrywide crises Indians had faced since Partition.

We weren't entirely alone in the second wave.

I remember Ashutosh Mishra from *India Today*, always one step ahead or behind me, reaching the cities and towns I had just entered or left. We nearly crossed paths in Buxar. There was also Swati Mishra from *Lallantop*, who navigated Uttar Pradesh in April, reporting from crematoriums and tracking the oxygen crisis. Sohit Mishra from NDTV reported from Mumbai and Salman Ravi, working with BBC Hindi, reported from Delhi.

I also recall Vinod Kapri's haunting documentary on migrant workers, late Danish Siddiqui's striking follow-up on the father-son photograph from the first wave and Barkha Dutt's unrelenting on-ground reporting through Mojo.

Then, the landscape of the media industry itself shifted.

Two years into the pandemic, independent YouTube channels began to flourish. There was an explosion of voices, perspectives and reportage. But long before this tsunami of YouTube channels, there were my colleagues—young women, spread across the country, travelling thousands of kilometres across both waves.

To come back to Durga Purwa in Sitapur district: when I asked the villagers, 'Virus ka naam suna hai?' (Have you heard of the virus?), a man called Sanjay said, 'Suna toh hai ki chuachhoot ki bimari hai. Lekin sheher ke logon ko ho rahi hai, gaon ke logon ko nahin.' (We have heard that this disease spreads through touch. But this is a city disease, village people won't catch it.)

That explained why most of them weren't covering their noses and mouths. They had bigger worries; all of the sons, husbands and fathers of the village hadn't returned yet.

Imran was a resident of Durga Purwa. His father had died in April but his brother, Kayyum, hadn't made it to the funeral. He was stranded in Delhi. He had left the village many moons ago to work at a tailoring shop in the national capital.

'Whenever we call him, he keeps crying. He tells us how scared he is of this outbreak in the city.' Imran further said that Kayyum was running out of food. His entire family were living their worst nightmares.

Across the river, in Nai Basti, the situation was even grimmer. There was no road or bridge that connected Nai Basti to the rest of the world. The village had no electricity, no phone towers and no kirana shops. Villagers had to walk more than four km to reach the river, and take a boat to reach Durga Purwa. From Durga Purwa, they would walk another ten to twelve km to reach banks and markets.

For both these villages, there was also a looming threat of floods. In just fifteen to twenty days, the river would flood their homes. Their tough lives worsened during the rainy season. They would prepare for months before monsoon, setting up temporary shelters to relocate to higher grounds.

The lockdown caught them unawares. They were dependent on wheat cultivation as their primary source of income, but as their access to the tehsil or the district headquarters got restricted, they were unable to travel to sell their harvest and it was piling up in their homes.

'The entire harvest will rot if we don't sell it on time,' Sanjay told us. They were facing an acute shortage of essential commodities. Many households had run out of tea, sugar, oil and salt.

Some families had started selling wheat in exchange for goods. When we were walking towards the river to catch a boat to Nai Basti, we found a few children with their mothers exchanging wheat for watermelons.

The boat was arranged for by the village head. The two people escorting us had also brought their bikes along so that we could reach the faraway Nai Basti on time and return to the river before sunset.

A few locals tagged along to save the money they would otherwise have to pay to the ferryman.

Once across the river, we were taken to Nai Basti on bikes. This was a small settlement; there was no panchayat bhawan, no government school and no Bolero parked outside the village head's house.

Now we understood why the villagers said that the virus was only killing people in the city and would never reach them. This was so remote an area that even the administration was unable to fully establish its presence there.

All this time I was careful to not take my mask off because I had a sore throat and no amount of hot water or Vicks lozenges were helping. I suspected it wasn't COVID but the result of stepping out of an air-conditioned car into the blazing heat of May every time we passed a group of migrants, bus stops or villages that I thought would make for powerful images. Several times a day, I'd ask Manish to stop the car and run out with my trusty iPhone X—which I had bought a year ago when I first started reporting from rural and small-town India.

Since 2019, I have clicked pictures, recorded videos, done the research and conducted interviews all on my own for most of my stories. This is to say that as reporters, we seamlessly transitioned from traditional cameras to mobile journalism and the COVID years played a crucial role in its evolution. This shift is what led to the phenomenal success of *Mojo Story*.

We spent a considerable amount of time with the villagers of Nai Basti, talking about COVID, the migrant exodus and the lockdown. After a while, a few of them started covering their noses and mouths with gamchchas.

I interviewed seventy-year-old Ramphal. He had two young sons: twenty-five–year–old Anil and nineteen-year-old Pramod. Both had left to work in an iron factory in Punjab a few years ago. In the last few weeks, a few migrants had started returning to surrounding villages, but Ramphal's sons were still stuck in Punjab. The factory had shut down, they were out of work. Fifty days into the lockdown, they had run out of money and food.

Ramphal broke down. 'We don't own a phone. We can only talk to our sons when our neighbours lend us their phones, that too, on the other side of the river where there is network. Only we know how we are spending our days. Our heart aches when we listen to both our sons weeping on the phone every time we call them.'

Ramphal had borrowed money to send to his sons; the debt was mounting on him.

'People in the village have stopped giving us money. The bank is far away from here. There is no vehicle that can take us there,' Ramphal lamented.

Ramphal ended the interview with, 'We have no idea if we will ever see our sons again.'

This assignment was turning out to be a series of heartbreaks for my colleagues and me. What could we tell the old man? We had no answers but to leave with an assurance that his sons would be back.

'Please deliver my message to sarkar (authorities).' He folded his hands as tears ran down his cheeks.

On our way to Sitapur from Nai Basti, we were stalled by a fierce windstorm that lasted close to 15-20 minutes. We halted under a huge banyan tree and opened our lunch boxes. The pooris packed by Sadhana Shukla tasted better than anything we had ever eaten.

We spent the night in the banquet hall with its homesick staff from Uttarakhand. Home was where everyone wanted to be.

THE LUCKNOW-GORAKHPUR HIGHWAY

On 11 May, before we started for Gorakhpur, CM Yogi Adityanath's home turf, we fulfilled our promise of eating a meal with the banquet hall's owner at his residence. We ate with him and his wife. We departed with filled stomachs and packed meals for our journey.

It should have taken us seven hours to traverse the 355 kms to Gorakhpur but it took much longer; there was a long line of migrants on the highway.

According to the Ministry of Road Transport & Highways, a total of 1.6 crore migrants reached their native places during the lockdown. Out of this, 63.19 lakh migrants were ferried by the Railways in 4,621 Shramik trains between May and August.[17] This means that 42,81,000 migrants either walked, cycled, boarded trucks, booked private buses or used tempos, and even thelas, to reach their villages. And thousands couldn't make it.

Between March and June, 81,385 road accidents were recorded, which resulted in 29,415 deaths.[18] But the Centre did not maintain separate data on the number of migrant deaths in such accidents.

The 42,81,000 migrants had names, faces and families. They were left to sleep hungry and die alone away from their roots.

Dinesh Jaiswal, a native of Basti district in Uttar Pradesh, along with his wife Maithili, made a four-day journey in an autorickshaw from Mumbai, mapping 1,500 kilometres. Manish, Bismee and I met the couple on 11 May on the Lucknow–Gorakhpur highway.

Dinesh had left for Mumbai to work in a glass factory ten years ago. Within two years of settling in, he had married Maithili. Their life took a serious hit because of the lockdown. First, the factory was shut down, then they exhausted their savings.

'I packed roti-bhaji but it lasted us only two days. Since then, we have been surviving on meagre amounts of food.' Maithili said that nothing mattered more to the couple than getting home fast.

They had three co-travellers who shared similar stories of joblessness, cash crunch and lack of food. They stopped at petrol pumps and public parks to rest at night before proceeding on their journey after dawn.

A group of six tailors from Delhi were facing similar hardships. Natives of UP and Bihar, they had worked in Delhi's Kapashera for years. The loss of jobs wasn't the only problem that migrants like them were facing. Their landlords had started demanding next month's rent.

'I am the only source of income for my family of six in Bihar. Our landlord kept asking us to pay rent (Rs 5,000). There was no way we could manage it,' said Rustom Miyan, one of the tailors.

He echoed the sentiments of the millions of migrants who had decided to leave cities after the lockdown was announced, 'I feel that people like us will die more from hunger than from COVID.'

Amruddin, another tailor from the group, said he got fed up of eating salt and roti for ten-fifteen days after they ran out of money.

'Six of us stayed in one room. If one of us got infected, we would all catch the virus. So, we left on our cycles. At least some of us will reach home if not all,' he said.

Jeet, also part of the group, said, 'Staying hungry in my village with my family works for me. I won't be alone in this crisis. We have suffered a lot in the city, so we are running away like this.'

They had decided to leave Delhi on 6 May. They cycled for 500–600 kilometres before finding a truck to board in Barabanki, UP. We climbed into the truck to see for ourselves how they were managing to travel for hundreds of kilometres sitting on iron rods, or on stones or sand, all of which would heat up badly in the sun.

This truck ride wasn't free; the tailors paid thousands to hitch the ride.

We came across another group of forty-four migrants travelling from Rajasthan's Alwar to Uttar Pradesh on a bus; each of them had had to pay 3,670 rupees for their seat.

Abdul Mallick, a construction worker, could not wait any longer when he heard that a bus was being arranged by a group of workers.

'My family immediately transferred some money to my account so I could board the bus,' he said.

Bus driver Ajit Kant explained why he was charging three times the normal fare. Getting an interstate travel permit issued by the district collector in Alwar had cost him. The e-pass on the windshield of the bus, which ensured their smooth passage at every checkpoint and police barricade, cost some money too he claimed.

He was lying. State governments were not charging anything for issuing e-passes to the buses ferrying the migrants. In fact, just that day, the Gehlot government in Rajasthan had relaxed the travel rules and allowed inter-district and intra-district travel without a pass between 7 a.m. and 7 p.m.

In any case, the high fare hadn't stopped those forty-four migrants from taking this bus home, even though the trust between the mighty state and the migrants was broken.

SANT KABIR NAGAR

A photograph that I clicked on NH 28 became a symbolic representation of the migrant exodus. Five years later, we still use it as a feature in our COVID stories. The picture showed a group of seven migrants packed in the back of a stone-filled truck. There was barely any space for them amidst the stones. Yet they got on it along with three cycles. They tied two cycles to the wooden planks attached to the truck, while a migrant held the third for the entirety of their journey.

The sun was about to set on 11 May and we were not very far from Gorakhpur. My phone rang. It was Sangeeta. She had checked with many hotels in Gorakhpur, but none could take us in.

'They are citing strict lockdown guidelines,' she told me.

Entering the city, exiting and driving around Gorakhpur town while documenting the crisis wasn't going to be easy. There were many screening camps. It was a lot more organised, but a lot messier too. Gorakhpur being the chief minister's home turf, the local administration's scrutiny was heightened and lockdown restrictions were stricter across all aspects. Enforcing stringent rules, however, created further chaos at this time, turning the shutdown into an increasingly messy affair.

We started looking for motels along the highway, on the outskirts of Khalilabad, the headquarter of Sant Kabir Nagar district.

After a while, we came by a deserted yet decent-looking hotel. The receptionist allowed us in. Yet again, we were the only guests. At this point, the Basti, Sant Kabir Nagar and Gorakhpur districts had started reporting positive cases of migrants who had travelled from either Mumbai or Surat. They were mostly asymptomatic. We were being extra cautious while conducting interviews inside buses and on trucks because most migrants covered their mouths and noses with only handkerchiefs or gamchhas—not nearly as effective as N-95 masks.

As soon as migrants spotted us on the highway, they would crowd around our car. They wanted to be heard. How could one follow social distancing, maintain the 'do gaz ki duri' here? On a few occasions, we drove past hordes of people. They would rush towards us, and when we slowed down, they would plead with us to give a lift to the tired, ailing members of their group. They were not just a handful of people. As far as our eyes could see, there would be thousands of migrants on the road. While our car could only accommodate one more person; along with Manish, Bismee and I, the vehicle was crammed with luggage, bags of medicines, sanitisers, as well as the video kit. Some of them would peek inside the car and then go quiet. Only after making sure that we couldn't really help, would they let us go. Other than offering water bottles and some biscuits, we had nothing to offer to them.

I often wondered if we had to take one person along, who it would be. Everyone was wounded. You couldn't possibly choose one over the other. Besides, we could be booked by the state for grave negligence if any of us got infected and drove in close proximity to other people. We could be accused of spreading the virus and rounded up.

We were scared for our own lives as much as we feared for theirs. The virus could just as easily take us down as the people we were trying to help. As the wheels of our car moved forward, we left those helpless eyes behind.

My throat was getting worse, and I could sense a fever coming. That night in the hotel, I read obsessively about coronavirus and its symptoms. I started to panic. Where had I gone wrong? I was wearing the mask religiously; I was bathing in scalding hot water in the middle of May; I washed my hair every night; I was regularly sanitising my phone, slippers, shoes, mic, etc. That night I even sanitised the tiny earrings I wore. I couldn't sleep. I wept. I couldn't let my editors down. They had placed their faith in me. Would we be asked to return if I tested positive? What if we were quarantined here in UP?

I called Bismee to my room and confided in her. She dialled her doctor in Delhi. I also made a call to Praveen; he connected me with a doctor who was treating COVID patients in Delhi. I spoke to both doctors. I was panicking because I was aware of the death toll. On 11 May 2020, India had reported the biggest single-day spike of 4,213 new cases. We had had a total of 67,152 COVID cases by then.[19] Of these 20,917 were recovered cases. But there were 2,206 patients who had not made it. My panic also stemmed from the fear of the amount of social media trolling I would be subjected to if people found out that I was infected; the troll army would label me as a superspreader, they would issue threats.

I took the medicines the doctors prescribed and gargled. I felt better the next morning. We were on our seventh day of reporting. Manish and I left to visit the district hospital, quarantine centres and a few red zones.

The Ministry of Home Affairs (MHA) had classified containment areas into:[20]

- Red zone: a COVID hotspot with a large number of positive cases
- Orange zone: an area with a limited number of cases in the past but no surge in positive cases
- Green zone: an area with no positive cases

If a locality did not report any new COVID cases in twenty-eight days, it would be moved to the green zone.

Red zones were barricaded and police were deployed outside them. No outsiders were let in. The movement of the people living inside was heavily restricted.

We couldn't go inside the red zones, so I asked Manish to drive some distance on the Lucknow–Gorakhpur highway. There was a wave of migrants marching towards Khalilabad. We found out that they were headed to Sant Kabir Nagar District Jail. The jail was close to the highway.

Since some of the jails were under construction, the administration had turned them into COVID-19 screening centres. Every migrant, who either walked or boarded a bus or a truck, had to get their temperature checked at these screening centres. If they had a fever, they would be placed in quarantine centres and released only after fourteen days. Those who passed the test could walk to their villages.

We crossed queues several kilometres long to reach the district hospital and the jail. The two buildings—the hospital and the jail—stood at a distance from each other but shared the same road. A long queue of migrants stretched along it. We saw a man fall out of the queue. A few people gathered around him but we didn't give it much thought; he was probably trying to jump the queue.

We went up to the main gate of the screening point and returned the same way. At the spot where the man had fallen out of queue, there was a lot of chatter going on.

The man wasn't there. The man who had stood behind him said that he had asked for water and collapsed. Probably a policeman had taken him to the district hospital.

This Sadar Hospital looked just the same as all the others we had been to along our journey—weather-beaten walls, littered surroundings, nondescript. I walked inside with a diary in one hand, a phone in another, a tight mask on my face and my hair covered with a gamchha.

I saw a few policemen outside the main ward, their face shields on, watching videos on their phones to kill time. At a distance, some families sat on the ground and on benches, their faces pale.

'Woh jo ek migrant laya gaya tha na, wo kidhar hai?' (Where is the migrant who was just brought here?) I asked the policemen. They pointed to a two-room set up. 'The Collector is sitting there. Go ask him dir命ctly,' they said and went back to their phones.

I walked into one of the rooms. District Magistrate Ravish Gupta sat there in a PPE kit. Two other officials were there too. The premises were guarded by several policemen.

I began by introducing myself. He offered a chair and asked, 'Will you have tea?' I politely declined.

I enquired about the migrant who had fainted at the screening queue. The Collector said, 'He died on the spot. A postmortem is being conducted. A COVID test has been done because he was travelling from Mumbai.'

One of his sons had been traced.

'He has been informed about the death. For further information, please visit the police headquarters.' One of the two officials got up and gave me directions to the police headquarters.

We reached the police headquarters in a few minutes. I met ASP (assistant superintendent of police) Asit Srivastava who gave me the details of the man. His name was Ram Kripal and he was sixty-eight. The police had recovered nothing except a painkiller and a bottle of water from his person.

'His son Surinder is on his way,' Srivastava said. The story wouldn't end here. The police would trace the truck that he had boarded from Mumbai, then the co-passengers who went their way after getting off the same truck would be traced. The administration would wait for their COVID test results before deciding on the plan of action.

I took Surinder's number from Srivastava and headed to the hospital again. As I was entering from the side entrance, I saw a young man in a blue PPE kit sitting on the stairs that lead to the restroom, and crying.

'Are you Surinder?' I asked him. I had called the phone number that the police had given me, but nobody had responded. He nodded. But he kept sitting on the stairs.

He couldn't stop crying.

For the next ten minutes, we waited there for his father's body to be released. The administration had given him the PPE kit and gloves. The ambulance driver was also given a PPE kit.

Two men in PPE kits holding a big container of sanitiser walked up to us.

I called my managing editor, Y.P. Rajesh, to share the story of this migrant who couldn't make it home. As soon as Y.P. gave me the go-ahead, I called Bismee to get ready because we were going to cover the last rites of Ram Kripal. Manish went to the hotel to pick up Bismee and get the video kit.

By then I had introduced myself to Surinder and requested him to allow us to attend the last rites.

Ram Kripal was a resident of Haiser village in Sant Kabir Nagar district. He had two sons, Surinder and Mahinder, and a daughter, besides his wife in the family.

Twenty years ago, he had left for Mumbai to work in a paint polish factory. He could only manage to visit his home once a year. He wasn't one of the few lakh migrants who started to walk just after the announcement of the lockdown. He had waited until his patience ran out; the lockdown was extended two times, then three, until he became restless and decided to start his 1,600 kilometre-long journey from Mumbai. He was only thirty kilometres from home when he collapsed.

'We asked him to wait for the Shramik train but he shunned the idea as he desperately wanted to be with us,' Surinder told me.

His corpse was laid in a black plastic body bag for his final journey. Two men in PPE suits sprayed the body with sanitiser and left.

By now, Surinder's tears had dried up. He sat next to his father in the ambulance, which was escorted by three government vehicles as it exited the hospital and made its way to Bhidhar Shamshan ghat, a cremation site on the Ghaggar river. His family and acquaintances had gathered outside his village to receive the body, but the administration informed Surinder about the change of plan as they feared Ram Kripal's body could still be infectious. His village wasn't far from the cremation ground, some of the villagers jumped on their tractors and came immediately. Ram Kripal could not be home even in death.

At the riverbank, there were several policemen with face shields and three district administration officials fully covered in PPE suits. Two men from the Dom caste (cremators)—Kamal Babu Chaudhary and Munna Chaudhary (names changed to protect identity)—waited to perform the cremation; this had been their job for the last thirty years. The officials had brought two PPE kits for them too.

'Are you afraid?' I asked them. They said, 'Why would we be afraid? We have been doing this all our lives.'

This was my first time in a cremation ground. As a young girl growing up in a Haryanavi village, I was always discouraged by the women in my family from stepping out into the street whenever a funeral procession passed. I had never seen the cremation ground in my village, I was forbidden from going there. We were told horror stories of spirits and dead men walking. Now, witnessing Ram Kripal's funeral, was overwhelming.

Ram Kripal's family arrived on a tractor that was stopped half a kilometre away from the pyre. His wife wept and pleaded that she be allowed to see him for the last time, but only Surinder was allowed near the pyre to perform the last rites.

One of the three district officials who stood near the pyre wearing a PPE suit and getting ready for a photo was the BDO (block development officer). I couldn't resist asking him if the wife could be given a PPE suit and allowed a moment to say her goodbyes.'

'We don't have enough PPEs. So I cannot take the risk,' he said.

The twenty or so policemen on the job got their pictures clicked from various angles, and the officials insisted on some candid shots. Surinder squatted in a corner waiting for the photo op to get done. Soon, he and the two Doms were allowed to do their job.

The photos appeared in the local newspapers the next day despite there being no reporters on the site apart from Bismee and me. The officials had supplied the photos to the newspapers with headlines declaring that some officials were performing their duties in PPE kits.

After the funeral, Surinder had sat down at some distance from the pyre, staring into the river. His trance hadn't lasted long though. The administration admitted him to a quarantine centre where he was to spend the next fourteen days.

The tractor's driver was asked to go back to the village, and we followed.

Ram Kripal's wife started breaking the bangles on her wrists as soon as she entered her street. She sat outside the house and recalled his last phone call to her. 'He called me up around 11 a.m. this morning after getting down from a truck and said he would be home soon. He asked me to wait for him ...'

The next morning, I received a call from Surinder. He said this mother had been put in a quarantine centre in the district hospital along with both his brothers

'Gareeb hona koi kasoor hai kya? Ek to pita-ji nahi rahe, upar se uthakar yahan patak diya hai. Kya maut ka dukh bhi nahi karne denge kya?' (Is it a crime to be poor? We lost our father, and now they have locked us here. Are we not even allowed to mourn?) Surinder was sobbing.

This decision taken by the administration was absurd. Ram Kripal's family hadn't been allowed near his body or the pyre. The funeral was attended by the three block officials, the two Doms, twenty odd policemen and us two journalists.

I told Surinder I would call him back. Then I called the Collector, who said this was done as a measure of 'extra precaution'.

The samples of three people who hadn't been allowed to see their loved one one last time were sent to BRD (Baba Raghav Das Medical College) hospital in Gorakhpur. During the first wave, only government medical colleges were equipped to conduct COVID tests.

Ram Kripal's report came two days later. He was COVID positive.

THE GORAKHPUR-GOPALGANJ BORDER

After a lonely breakfast, the three of us checked out of the desolate hotel on the morning of 13 May. This was the kind of loneliness Ram Kripal had wanted to escape.

Before entering the Gorakhpur–Gopalganj border, we registered our names and got ourselves screened. At each checkpoint, a team of healthcare workers would be sweating it out in their PPE suits, taking temperatures of everyone who wanted to pass..

A few kilometres away from this last checkpoint in Gorakhpur, there was a transit centre—one of the five entry points into Bihar. The five entry points were Gopalganj, Kaimur, Gaya, Buxar and Purnea. Those who came from Rajasthan, Punjab, Haryana, Delhi, Gujarat, etc. entered via Gopalganj. Travellers from northeastern states entered via Purnea. Migrants who came from the southern states entered through Gaya and Kaimur. These transit centres were chaotic spaces where lakhs of migrants would catch buses to the last mile home.

We managed to get to Gopalganj by evening. There weren't many hotels and we knew no one there, so we went straight to Gopalganj's SP (Superintendent of Police) Manoj Kumar Tiwari. He spoke to the Collector, Arshad Aziz, about our request to stay in circuit houses. Circuit houses are usually reserved for politicians and their staff, government administration officials or guests of the district administration.

But the circuit houses had also been shut due to the lockdown. The staff, including cooks, had left for their villages. We were lucky to be given rooms. They hadn't been cleaned for weeks. There was dust and bugs and lizards.

When we stepped out of the collectorate after meeting the SP and Collector, the main market was flooded with people. Apparently, whenever there was some relaxation in the curfew, people would rush to the market to buy groceries, vegetables, medicines, etc.

But when we visited the market in the evening, it was deserted. The local administrations in many parts of Bihar would relax the lockdown for a short while every day so that people wouldn't run out of essential goods.

We spent the night in the circuit house. On the morning of 14 May, we went to the transit centre. Nearly a lakh migrants had gathered in a radius of five kilometres. Dozens of healthworkers screened them one at a time. The area was packed with buses, ambulances, loudspeakers and water and packaged food stalls.

There wasn't an inch to stand on until a few buses left for their respective districts. As men ran from one bus to another, from one counter to another, women and children held onto each other under makeshift tents.

There were a few who could not find seats on the buses, so they left for their home districts on foot, dragging their luggage behind them.

Manish spotted a heavily pregnant woman in the crowd. Twenty-eight-year-old Rekha Devi was due any day now. Somebody had offered her a chair while her husband had gone to find a bus that would take them home. The tiny chair could barely contain her as she sat anxiously holding her belly. Manish called Bismee, they offered her water and found her a more comfortable place to sit.

Bismee ran towards me, we were having to shout at each other in order to be heard in that noise. Rekha had travelled 900 kms—from Noida to Gopalganj—partly on foot and then in a truck; and now she was in labour.

'Uska bachcha kabhi bhi ho sakta hai.' She might deliver anytime now, a female relative of Rekha Devi informed us.

Rekha needed to be hospitalised urgently but we'd have to navigate a crowd of thousands to get to an ambulance.

I tried calling the Collector and SP for help, but the calls went unanswered. I walked out of the tent and there they were, inspecting the site. Their guards wouldn't let me through, so I resumed calling until the SP answered. He promised to send an ambulance.

It wasn't easy to convince Rekha Devi's family of nineteen, who had all journeyed from Greater Noida and just wanted seats on a bus.

Her husband, thirty-two-year-old daily wage worker Sandeep, was looking for a bus that would take them to Supaul, 300 kilometres away from the transit centre. He blatantly refused to accept help.

'Bas ghar bhijwa deejiye. Raaste mein delivery kara lenge.' Just help us get home. We will manage the delivery on the bus, he kept saying.

At this point, I lost patience. Rekha was going to deliver her fifth child. She was already in labour and her water could break any time.

'Kyon jaan ke sath khel rahe hain? Raaste itne kharab hain, inki haalat bigad jayegi.' (Why are you risking her life? The roads are in bad shape, her situation can get worse.) I didn't give up.

The female relative who had heard me talking to the SP tried to bargain for seats on a bus from the administration; Rekha's husband too started requesting for the same so that they could take her home.

'I promise you that you will be dropped home. Please allow Rekha to go to a hospital first,' I insisted. The persuation worked. We followed the ambulance to the district hospital. Around 3 p.m., we returned to the circuit house.

An hour later, Manish drove me to the hospital again. I thought Rekha Devi must have delivered by now, so I would go arrange the bus for them. On the way, I bought some chips, biscuits and water bottles for Rekha's children. Once there, I couldn't find them in any of the wards.

Somebody guided me to the labour ward. Sandeep was sitting with his youngest daughter on his lap. Upon seeing me, he burst out crying. We came down to the parking area and I gave a packet of chips to his daughter.

'Pehle toh bharti nahin kiya ki Corona hoga. Phir bharti jaise taise karaya toh ab ilaaj nahi kar rahe hain ki baccha paanch din baad hoga. Nurse paas hi nahin aa rahi hai,' (First, they refused to admit her. Now they've admitted her but they aren't treating her because they think she might be infected. They say she will deliver in five days, and no nurse is coming near her), he told me.

In the labour room, nurses were engaged in file work. I came out and called the Collector again, and he called the medical superintendent.

A senior doctor was assigned to the case. Nurses rushed to Rekha's bed. I sat down on the bench next to Sandeep. Their extended family had stayed at the transit centre, waiting for the bus. Only Sandeep, his wife and one of the daughters had come to hospital.

'Are you her relative?' one of the nurses came out and asked me. I nodded, so she called me in. I was a bit nervous but I continued standing there.

'Collector sir called,' the nurse who had summoned me told the other two nurses in the labour room. They were in their forties and fifties and knew their job well.

'Aap yahin rahiye aur dekhiye ki hum kitne achche se delivery karte hain. Aap Collector sir ko bataana bhi.' (You stay here and observe how well we do it. Please let Collector sir know.)

It was a natural birth. This was my first time witnessing a child being born. I had goosebumps.

As she pushed, Rekha was too tired to even cry. The nurse ranted about the condition in which Rekha had been admitted.

'This is her fifth child. Her body is too weak to bear so many pregnancies. In such delays, women often don't make it,' one of the other nurses said.

At 5.45, a baby girl was born. Drenched in blood, she did not cry for a few seconds. When the nurses patted her back, she let out a loud cry.

In a span of seventy-two hours, I had seen a life end and a life begin. A cremation and a birth!

Growing up in a joint family, I remember a moment from my childhood. My aunt was pregnant with her sixth child. She had five daughters, two of whom didn't survive. One died shortly after birth, the other was taken before she could even enter the world. My mother and other women in the family often whispered behind my aunt's back that she had boiled and consumed a whole lot of carrot leaves, believing it would make her uterus too hot to hold the baby. Such DIY hacks are secretly used by Indian women to abort an unwanted child (more often than not, a girl child). The girl child's fate was sealed the moment her sex was determined. Haryana was infamous for its female foeticide rate.

The sixth child was a son. Hospital deliveries weren't the norm in our village back then. When my aunt went into labor, the children, including me, were sent outside. A midwife was called in. I ran to fetch my grandmother from the fields, telling her that my aunt was crying. My mother, too, was pulled away from her household chores.

We played in the courtyard, under the neem tree, oblivious to what was going on inside the dark room. All we could hear were cries. And then, suddenly, he was here.

That is my faintest memory of childbirth.

Birth, as shown in movies, is loud, dramatic. The cries of a mother, the first wail of a newborn, the celebratory 'Badhai ho, aap papa ban gaye'. But it isn't like that in real life. It is hours upon hours of intense labour pain—a near-death experience for a woman.

That day, the romanticism of childbirth, the one I had read about, the one I had seen, ended for me.

What I witnessed was a woman too numb, too exhausted to even cry.

But on the other side of this near-death experience, there is one sound a mother awaits: the first cry of her newborn. It is the moment that makes the suffering worth it, the sound that carries life itself. It is the most magical sound—as I experienced for myself when I gave birth to my daughter.

I was overjoyed until I broke the news to Sandeep who was waiting outside the labour room. When I informed him that it was a baby girl, he started howling like he had lost someone.

'Are you not happy that your wife and child are safe?'

'Ek toh garibi aur upar se paanch betiyaan. Inka dahej kahan se laaunga?' (I am poor, how will I arrange dowry for five daughters?)

I met the Collector later that evening to thank him for intervening and requested a bus to take the family to Supaul. A week later, while we were still on the highway, I got a call from Sandeep that they had safely reached home.

In November 2020, when Bihar voted in their assembly election, everyone wanted to see how the migrants would vote. Would their anguish guide their voting?

Sandeep returned to Greater Noida in September. His wife followed three weeks later with three of their children, leaving the other two behind with their grandparents. I met them in their 10 feet by 10 feet room in Parthala Market in Sector 122, Noida. They gave the state elections a miss. I asked them if they had forgotten what they went through in April and May. They said they hadn't.

'Nitish Kumar asked the migrants to stay wherever we were, while other states called their people back. Without a paisa in our pockets and ration in our homes, we were left to die. How can we forget and forgive him?' Migrants like Sandeep had lost faith in the state.

SITAMARHI

The story of Ram Kripal from UP was tied inextricably to the story of Sandeep and Rekha from Bihar. Their stories of death and birth reflected the experiences of millions of migrants in India.

Our assignment had taken us across 1400 km, but our journey to capture the realities of COVID was far from over. On the morning of 15 May, our tenth day on the road, we set off for Sitamarhi district, situated on the edge of India and Nepal and believed to be the birthplace of Sita. The district is also a part of Mithilanchal, a region that has a unique cultural identity within the state.

According to the 2011 census, 88.71 per cent of Sitamarhi district's people lived in villages—higher than the national average of 68.84 per cent. So only 11.29 per cent of the people in Sitamarhi lived in urban areas. Bihar has long been pushing for urbanisation, but has it made any progress to be able to join India's growth story of infrastructure boom and rapid urbanisation?

We had hoped to find some answers from the 2021 census. But the census got postponed due to COVID-19. The Centre had notified the *Gazette of India* in March 2019 that the exercise was to be carried out in two phases—housing census in 2020 and population enumeration in 2021. However, delays pushed it further to 2022, then 2023 and now, Union Minister Kishan Reddy has said that the census may take place in 2026 to align with the delimitation schedule.[21]

In a surprising turn of events, the central government declared in April 2025 that it would also conduct a caste census in India.[22] All eyes are on how this will unfold. Meanwhile, Bihar has already taken the lead, having carried out its own caste survey.

After a 200-kilometre journey via Muzaffarpur, we arrived at the district headquarters by evening. Yet again, no accommodation. I called SP Anil Kumar and requested him to seek the Collector's permission for us to lodge in the circuit house for a day.

This circuit house was beautiful; its walls were adorned with Madhubani art. We waited at the gate, which had been shut for over a month, until a guard showed up and let us in.

After freshening up, we headed to the SP's residential office for a meeting. He gave us the data on returned migrants, the arrangements made for them and lockdown enforcement strategies—all of which sounded familiar. But we knew there were stories that were hidden, stories that were beyond the checkpoints, the police barricades and the curfew hours.

Back at the circuit house, the guard offered us snacks while Manish strolled around town to find food.

The next morning, Manish and I headed to a panchayat called Singhwahini in Sonbarsa block. In 2016, Singhwahini had gained recognition by electing a woman mukhiya—Ritu Jaiswal, which had made the national media train all their lenses on this tiny panchayat of seven villages on the Indo–Nepal border. Ritu Jaiswal was making headlines for her work as a woman mukhiya. Her husband, Arun Kumar, is an ex-IOFS (Indian Ordinance Factories Service) official from the 1995 batch. He had voluntarily retired from the service and opened a civil services coaching institute in Patna.

Besides being a mukhiya, Ritu was also affiliated with the Janata Dal United (JDU) party. She parted ways with them in September 2020 and joined the Rashtriya Janata Dal (RJD), fought the 2020 assembly election from Parihar but lost by 1569 votes. She was then appointed state president of the women's wing of the RJD. In 2021, when the panchayat elections were held again, her husband contested for the mukhiya's seat and secured it.[23]

Singhwahini was situated twenty-five kilometres away from the district headquarters. We met Ritu Jaiswal at the panchayat. She gave me a tour and introduced me to many women whose husbands had migrated to other cities. The COVID-19 lockdown and the migrant workers' crisis had worsened the lives of these women. For example, in Sitamarhi, the men who returned home had no savings or income to support their families, while the men who were still on the road or stranded in other states needed money. The women took it upon themselves to send them money for their survival or return.

The shift of the economic burden on women led to many illegally borrowing from moneylenders at high interest rates. The Bihar Money Lenders Act of 1974 prohibits private moneylenders who are not registered with the state government from lending money. But the women, despite its illegality and the five-times-higher interest rates, had no other choice.

I went to three villages in Singhwahini panchayat—Jankinagar, Malhatola and Kaharwa—to look into this troubling trend. (Tolas are caste-based segregated areas in a village.)

Indu Devi, fifty-five, had three sons—Ashok, Alok and Santosh—all daily-wage construction workers stranded in Punjab. This family in Malha tola had nine members, including three children between ages two and six. Her husband had died many years ago—she had no recollection of how long it had been.

Not only had the burden of supporting the family fallen on her shoulders, but Indu Devi also had to arrange money for Alok's seven-month pregnant wife Ragini's delivery. She didn't know when her sons would return and whether they would have any money when they did. 'I have no land, the only income I have is from selling cow milk, and the goats I had bought by taking a loan under the Jeevika programme (part of the Bihar Rural Livelihoods Promotion Society) before the lockdown.

'I have to send money to my sons. Their lala (contractor) has been asking them to pay rent. I have taken a loan of 50,000 rupees at an interest of monthly 5 per cent, out of which I have sent 20,000 to my sons, and kept the rest to feed the family, and for Ragini's delivery.' She wouldn't let her children die of hunger even if she had to borrow money one more time.

When I asked her if her sons had tried to return on the central government-run Shramik trains, she said she didn't understand the new government scheme.

After the interview, she resumed her daily chores and I left to meet Bindu Devi in Jankinagar. She had a similar story. She had taken a loan of 15,000 rupees. Her husband was stuck in Muzaffarpur, where he worked in a fabric shop. She had been sending money so he could recharge his phone and buy food. She had taken a loan at 6 per cent monthly interest.

The state had to step in to rescue the women from their mounting debt. So, the panchayats were given the task of making masks under the Panchayat Nidhi Scheme. The district administration was instructed to purchase the masks from the panchayats at the rate of twenty rupees per mask. Bindu Devi was one of an army of women who stitched masks on sewing machines.

Apart from employing women to manufacture masks, the Bihar government also gave a 1,000 rupees each from the Prime

Minister's Relief Fund to 20 lakh people. Bihar's then Information Minister and a JDU MLC, Neeraj Kumar, told me that the government would, for the next two months, provide ration to the migrant workers who had returned to the state.

After I finished the women's debt story, Ritu Jaiswal offered to take me to the Nepal border for another story.

That evening, we met A.K. Jhakkar of the fifty-first battalion of the Sashastra Seema Bal (SSB). The Indo–Nepal border in Sitamarhi district runs through open fields, extending from Bairgania to Sursand for about eighty km. Since the announcement of lockdown, the SSB and police personnel posted at local border outposts had been intercepting migrants trying to cross over. There are no shelter homes in Sitamarhi, so these workers were placed in quarantine centres.

I met Raja Maheshwari, a migrant worker from Nepal, in the Bela Machhpakauni quarantine centre. He had come to India in March and found a job at a construction site in Bihar's Sasaram. He was just starting to settle in when the pandemic brought everything to a standstill.

So, on 15 April, Maheshwari and twenty other Nepalese workers started walking back to their homeland. But India and Nepal had both sealed their borders by then; the group of twenty-one migrant workers were caught by Nepal Police and handed over to India.

Of the thousands of Nepalis who had worked in different parts of India and travelled long distances to return to Nepal during lockdown, hundreds were stranded at the border—at least 300 at the Sitamarhi border alone. They remained stranded until June because the Nepalese government failed to arrive at a decision.

The International Labour Organisation published a paper that said there was no official record of how many Nepali workers were in India, but the National Labour Force Survey estimated it to be 587,646. Most of them worked in the informal sector, earning daily wages mainly in agriculture and construction. Since they had no formal employment contracts or benefits, their employers did not provide them with food, accommodation or healthcare.

At the Bela Macchpakauni quarantine centre, Chawdhary, a daily wage worker from Nepal had been stranded for over twenty days.

'I left Delhi on foot and got on a truck at Badarpur. When I reached Sitamarhi to cross over into Nepal, the police brought me here,' he said. Despite having spent fourteen days in quarantine, he wasn't allowed to leave.

'Why didn't you stay back in Delhi?' I asked him. He explained that his landlord was pressuring him to pay rent and he had no money to pay.

A.K. Jhakkar, who headed the team that stopped the first batch of seventeen Nepali workers returning from Haryana and Noida on 31 March at the Kanhwa border outpost said it was easy to recognise those who were going to cross the border.

'We keep interrogating people on the border. If someone says they have come to see their farm, we know they are Indians. Nepali migrants have a weary look on their faces, they look drained from the journey. We explain to them that they can't leave for Nepal because the borders are closed,' he said.

Thousands of migrants were held up at the Indo–Nepal border for more than forty days.

Sitamarhi's SP, Anil Kumar said he had brought up the matter with the Ministry of Home Affairs (MHA) and the Ministry of External Affairs (MEA) many times but the district administration was still waiting for an update from the central government.

'Until they tell us, we have no power. The lockdown has also held up many Indian workers in Nepal.'

My colleague Nayanima Basu, who reported on the MEA, later found out that the Nepal border was not the only one where thousands were stranded for months, but also the Bhutan and Bangladesh borders. The migrants would not receive any help until the countries on both sides of the border removed restrictions.

Manish and I returned from the Indo-Nepal border to the circuit house just before 9 p.m. Bismee was waiting for us. We had to leave for Katihar in the northeastern region of Seemanchal, Bihar, that night—a long journey of over 350 kilometers that would take us seven-eight hours.

We spent the night of 17 May in the car. We were travelling from a northwestern district to a northeastern district of Bihar to cover different regions and their problems.

KATIHAR

We chose to travel at night, wanting to use the daylight for reporting. It was surely risky to travel at night. Just Manish and us, two women driving on highways. We could get waylaid, robbed or assaulted, and as women, we were exposed to the possibility of sexual violence.

Bismee and I were both on our period. We were sleep-deprived and exhausted. We were worried about how we would manage to change our pads on the way. We thought of using the petrol pump toilets or the highway dhabas, but all the places were packed with migrants who had stopped to rest at night. We tried a few dhabas that looked upscale, but the washrooms were so filthy that we were afraid of getting infected. We ultimately decided to go behind the trees on the sides of the highway. Bismee watched my back when I changed, and I did the same for her.

When we received the 2020 Ramnath Goenka Award for Excellence for our coverage of the migrant exodus and the lockdown, and *The Indian Express* reporters asked us about the challenges we faced during the assignment, I mentioned the difficulty of finding clean toilets to change pads. On this, some people commented that women should not take up such assignments when they are so fragile.

During my reporting assignments, I have talked to many policewomen who are sent to protest sites or for investigations in faraway places—assignments that involve travel. They often say that they avoid drinking water so that they don't have to use public toilets while on the job. This is a reality for many women who must step out to work.

Of course, we faced many other challenges when we were covering the pandemic, but Bismee and I chose the platform the Ramnath Goenka Award gave us to raise the point that public infrastructure needs to be women-friendly, and public toilets are a big part of it

Manish kept his promise—we were at the Katihar Railway Junction by 8 a.m. The Katihar Railway division serves Bihar and West Bengal and also connects them with the northeastern states of India. It is one of the five railway divisions under the Northeast Frontier Railway zone of Indian Railways.

This was our twelfth day on the road. Bismee and I had managed to get some sleep. Manish was thoroughly exhausted because he had been driving all night. We needed somewhere to rest for a bit, but we did not know anyone in the town.

After parking our car in front of the railway station, Manish went to freshen up somewhere. I walked to the platforms. People poured in every hour, and were then led to different buses. I was taking pictures when a group of men started catcalling and passing lewd comments at me. Frustrated, I left and got in the car.

I called Collector Kanwal Tanuj and told him that we needed a place to stay. He refused saying an MP was staying in the circuit house. So, Bismee and I tried our contacts. Someone from Delhi connected me to a local politician who wanted to contest in the upcoming assembly elections. I won't name him because eventually he did not get the ticket, but he said that he would call a few hotel owners to see if they could arrange something for us.

But soon, Collector Kanwal Tanuj called back asking us to go to the circuit house. Once there, we met Dulal Chandra Goswami, the JDU (Janata Dal United) MP from Katihar's Lok Sabha seat. During our stay, he would often chat with us during meals and ask us about our coverage. Usually, MPs and MLAs who are in their constituencies have no time for long conversations, they have a long queue of constituents seeing counsel or asking for help. Since we were in lockdown, the MP did not have many visitors.

On 18 May, we visited the village and panchayat level quarantine centres in two blocks of Katihar—Manihari (close to the Jharkhand border) and Barsoi (near the West Bengal border).

The Bihar government had divided their quarantine centres into block, panchayat and village levels. At the block level shelters, migrants coming back from Delhi, Maharashtra and Gujarat were quarantined; those coming from West Bengal, Haryana, Tamil Nadu and Uttar Pradesh were put in panchayat level centres; and people coming back from other states were accommodated at village level quarantine centres.

Sanjay Kumar, who was then the principal secretary of Health, explained this segregation when I spoke to him. 'Delhi has the highest number of COVID-19 cases among migrant workers, followed by Maharashtra, West Bengal and Gujarat. This is what we've observed in Bihar.'

Most schools in the village had been converted into quarantine facilities. In some villages, the migrants' families would cook meals for them and leave them at the gates. In some quarantine centres, the administration provided ration and other essentials for the migrants to cook their own meals. Soon, they started distributing dignity kits that contained sixteen items, including combs, soaps, buckets, mosquito nets, bed sheets, etc. Many schools had no electricity, so the migrants spent nights under mosquito nets or with Odomos slathered on their bodies.

But it was tough to kill time. They were barely a few metres away from their homes and yet so far. At some schools, the village heads appointed a few men as guards to keep an eye on the migrants. The observance of social distancing and quarantine was important, but the way the migrants had been stuffed into these centres meant that those rules could not protect the poor.

The story that could not be told was about the many ways in which rural India copes with crises, and how immense the distance is between its people and those of us who read these stories in the papers is.

PURNEA-BHAGALPUR

Girindra Nath Jha, a landowner from Purnea, Bihar, was a journalist in Delhi for some years before he returned to his hometown and opened Chanka Residency, a two-bedroom set up on a vast farm with hundreds of Kadamba trees and a pond in his native village Chanka, twenty-five km away from Purnea. Many journalists from New Delhi toured the place during the election season.

Jha had been following our coverage of Bihar and dropped a message when he saw that we were in an adjoining district. We met him outside his residence in Purnea on 19 May. He was telling us about his writing on rural life, sharing his insights on the region, when we were notified of a tragic road accident that had killed nine migrant workers in Naugachia, Bhagalpur.

Jha joined us on the assignment.

It took us two hours to reach the scene of the accident. All we saw there were torn shoes, ripped clothes and remnants of food. The truck that the workers had been travelling on was loaded with iron bars and other construction materials. It now lay in a ditch where it had fallen after veering in an effort to avoid a collision with a bus full of migrants on National Highway 31.

Ambho village, which was near the highway, had woken up to a gruesome sight. The sarpanch had alerted the police as soon as he got to know.

'It was between five and six in the morning. The workers got trapped under the iron rods on which they had been sitting earlier,' said Manju, a forty-five-year-old woman, who was one of the first to reach the spot.

People tried to retrieve the bodies but they were lodged firmly under the iron rods. A crane was summoned to remove the rods and extricate the bodies.

Matwari Singh, another eyewitness who lived just a 100 metres away from the accident site, said that he was the first one to spot the truck. Those who had witnessed the horrific scene were shaken.

We hurried to the sub-divisional government hospital where the bodies were brought—all pronounced dead-on-arrival—and waited outside the mortuary, where identification was underway.

Six of them were identified: Jalim Miya, Mohammed Hasim and Nurjahan Miya hailed from Bettiah district; the other three—Gushan Miya, Mohammed Rustom and Shaukat Ali—were from Motihari district. They were still over eight hours away from their homes. They made their final journey home in ambulances escorted by police cars.

These people had started from Kolkata on bicycles six days ago, and had boarded the truck at some point in their journey

The bus they collided with had about twenty to twenty-five migrants on board; five of them had sustained injuries. They left for their homes a few hours later.

Meanwhile, the local police were chasing the drivers who had both fled the scene.

After a spate of similar accidents, the Bihar government requested all migrant workers to refrain from travelling on foot, or on rail tracks or trucks. They also announced a compensation of four lakh rupees for the families of those who had lost their lives in such accidents.

We dropped Girindra Nath Jha to his house on our way back to Katihar. But before we bid him farewell, he took us to the Purnea collectorate and introduced us to the then district magistrate, Rahul Kumar. Kumar told us about the sheer magnitude of the crisis and the administrative challenges it posed. All four of us were masked, so we didn't even have tea.

PATNA

Manish's wife is Muslim; his children kept urging him to return home for Eid. Bismee too wanted to be back with her family for the festivities. I wanted to return to Delhi too; the fatigue was unbearable.

On 20 May, we left Katihar in the morning and reached Patna by evening for the last leg of our assignment. My health was worsening by the day. I suffered a heatstroke and got really sick. A friend had once told me to get raw mangoes, boil them and apply the mashed pulp on my forehead and on my soles to prevent a heat stroke. So, the next day, Manish went looking for raw mangoes and returned hours later. 'I had to scour the whole city to find them,' he said, jokingly.

Like all big cities, Patna was under a strict lockdown. Sangeeta found us a hotel on Frazer Road at the Dak Bungalow Crossing, in the heart of Patna. It was in an old building that also had a newspaper office in it. The place was deserted. Even the Patna Secretariat was shut. There were police barricades in many places. Bihar had reported a total of 1,900 positive COVID-19 cases that day.

The locality with all the MLAs' residences was also very quiet. The political leaders had changed their routines. There were no rallies, programmes or meetings being held. There were no queues outside their gates; no OB vans outside the party offices of the RJD, the JDU, the Congress, or the BJP on Veer Chand Patel Marg.

However, the leaders who held cabinet portfolios were making calls and attending video conferences with the CM.

We called many people to get updates but most of our calls went unanswered. Still, we managed to meet BJP MLA Dr Prem Kumar, the Minister for Agriculture, Animal Husbandry and Fisheries, and JDU MLC Neeraj Kumar, the Minister for Information and Public Relations. They gave us their views on the situation in the state, mostly what they were already saying on social media platforms.

When I interviewed Tejashwi Yadav, he claimed that the migrant workers had returned to Bihar after months of hardship, but the government wasn't able to handle the influx. He slammed the Bihar government for its lax approach to COVID testing and the lack of development in Bihar's health infrastructure under Nitish Kumar's rule.

He said that even Haryana was doing much better than Bihar in testing and saving its people, a remark that wasn't necessarily based on facts.

He expressed his suspicion over the transfer of IAS Sanjay Kumar, former principal secretary of the health department, amidst the surge in cases in the state. He alleged that Sanjay Kumar was removed because he did not bow down to the government's 'lobby of bureaucrats' and 'dictatorship'.

He said that Sanjay Kumar had suspended the head of the microbiology department in Patna's Nalanda Medical College and Hospital, who happened to be a close relative of Nitish Kumar's, and that had angered the Chief Minister. Sanjay Kumar never spoke about his abrupt transfer though.

On 23 May 2020, we started back for New Delhi, driving over a 1,000 kilometers in twenty-four hours. We took turns sleeping at petrol stations along the way. I was still quite sick and made it through the journey relying on ORS.

On May 24, we arrived in Delhi after a long assignment, reporting dozens of stories of pain, hunger, death, debt and fatigue. Of the numerous stories of lockdown and migrants that we became witness to, we were able to tell only a few. Many more went untold.

One story that really captured the national attention,, though I wasn't the first one to break it, was that of Jyoti Kumari. A teenager from Darbhanga, she had ridden a bicycle, then boarded a truck, with her injured father, Mohan Paswan, from Gurugram to Darbhanga in nine days, covering a distance of 1,200 kilometres.

A few days after she reached her village Sirhulli in Darbhanga, the story of Jyoti's incredible grit and resilience made her a national hero. A photograph of her with her father on the cycle became a symbol of the struggles that migrant workers and their families faced during the lockdown. She was given the alias 'Cycle Girl of Bihar'.

Ivanka Trump, the US President's daughter and senior advisor, praised Jyoti's act as a 'beautiful feat of endurance and love that has captured the imagination of the Indian people'. *The New York Times* described her as a 'lionhearted girl' who inspired a nation.[24]

Her heroism overshadowed the story of her father's migration and the reason why she cycled across north India.

Jyoti's father, Mohan Paswan, had left his village, Sirhulli, in 1996 to find work in Delhi. He had worked as an e-rickshaw driver in Gurugram for many years. His wife, Phoolo Devi, had been an Anganwadi cook for eight years in Darbhanga, Bihar. Together, they earned Rs 11,000–Rs 12,000 per month to support their family of five children.

On 26 January, 2020, Mohan's life took an unexpected turn when he was injured in an accident. His wife, son-in-law and Jyoti rushed to Gurugram by train on 30 January to care for him. While his wife and son-in-law returned to Bihar in February, Jyoti stayed behind.

For Jyoti, it was her first time experiencing a big city. But before she could fully grasp the new world around her, a nationwide lockdown was announced in March.

'We both got stuck in Gurugram,' Mohan told me.

As the days passed, their landlord began demanding rent, pushing the father-daughter duo into a desperate situation. With no other option, Jyoti made a bold decision—she would cycle home with her father.

'The landlady even disconnected our electricity,' Jyoti recalled. 'I pleaded with her to let us stay for just one more day, promising we would leave the next morning.'

With 500 rupees from her family's Jan Dhan account, she bought a second-hand cycle—their only means of escape. On 7 May, they set off from Gurugram, peddling towards their village in Darbhanga, covering hundreds of kilometres.

The journey was gruelling. A truck driver offered them a ride for part of the way, but not everyone was kind. 'Most truck drivers demanded 3,000-4,000 rupees,' Mohan said.

Back in their village, Jyoti's family tried to stop her from cycling. 'Her safety was at risk because she was a young girl,' her sister Pinky Paswan said. 'How could she cycle among crowds of men on the roads?'

But Jyoti refused to listen. She left Gurugram in a hurry, making only one phone call before departing. For nine nights, Pinky and their mother Phoolo Devi lived in fear.

Yet, what Mohan and Jyoti witnessed on the road was far worse than their own fears—millions of migrants walking on foot, carrying the burden of their meagre belongings, searching for a way home. 'At least we had an old cycle,' Mohan had told me. 'Some people were more helpless than us.'

A year later, in May 2021, Mohan Paswan died following a cardiac arrest during the second wave of COVID-19.

Despite the hardships, Jyoti remained determined to continue her studies. When I interviewed her in 2020, she expressed her dream of going back to school. That's when Darbhanga's district magistrate, S.M. Thiyagrajan stepped in, ensuring she was enrolled in Class 9.

'Jyoti told us she wanted to study and take part in cycle races,' Thiyagrajan told me.

Her story captured the nation's attention. RJD leader Tejashwi Yadav and former Bihar Chief Minister Rabri Devi offered to sponsor her education and wedding, and get a job for her father.[25]

Lok Janshakti Party MP Chirag Paswan pledged to support her studies.[26, 27]

Even Union Minister Late Ram Vilas Paswan referred to her as 'the modern-day Shravan Kumar', the mythological figure who carried his blind parents on his shoulders.[28]

Union Sports Minister, Kiren Rijiju, promised her a spot in Delhi's National Cycling Academy[29], and the founder of Super 30, Anand Kumar, offered to fund her education.

For some time, Jyoti remained in the spotlight. She even signed a film called *Aatmanirbhar*, in which she was to play herself. But soon, the cameras stopped rolling.

Her life faded from public memory.

She had some good moments in 2021, becoming the brand ambassador for an anti-drug abuse programme in Bihar and receiving the Pradhan Mantri Rashtriya Bal Puraskar on India's 72nd Republic Day. She was one of thirty-two children who won the award and even had a virtual chat with Prime Minister Narendra Modi.[30]

But four years have passed since that moment of glory, and Jyoti still hasn't been able to join a college. The help has stopped coming in.

Her dreams of studying further remain unfulfilled.

2

Between the Two Waves

By the time we returned from our assignment, Delhi had transformed. Traffic being minimal on the road for weeks, the air outside felt fresh. The sky wasn't choked with smog; it wasn't grey as before. Photographs from that year look like postcards from a different world. The skies were painted in the brightest blues, dotted with cotton ball clouds.

The lockdown was lifted across the country. But it didn't happen all at once. Not in the way it had been locked down in one swipe. The reopening unfolded slowly—in measured, carefully planned ways—month by month, stretching until the end of the year.

June brought some movement. One of the first things permitted was domestic air travel. Restaurants and religious places reopened in areas where cases weren't actively reported. Night curfews were lifted in July.

August marked the seventy-fourth year of India's independence. The guest list for flag hoisting at the Red Fort was reduced to a fourth; only 4,000 invitees attended the ceremony. In the following month, metro lines resumed operations, with designated gates to manage crowds and enforce the new normal. Schools and cinemas too came back to life, cautiously, with limited attendance.

In November and December, the Centre loosened its grip, allowing states to set their own pace and rules for normalcy. Yet nationwide SOPs remained in place: no gatherings of more than a hundred people, mandatory masks and compulsory COVID-19 testing.

In the media industry, story pitches began to diversify. Politics re-entered the frame, along with everything that had existed before—it's good, it's bad and it's unresolved. Politics, in truth, had never left. It had simply shifted to revolve around the virus. At *ThePrint*, the newsroom never fully transitioned to working from home. Most of us, from editors to those on the video team and the desk, continued coming in. As for reporters, we were embedded in the physical newsroom soon after returning from far-flung corners of the country.

Many of us believed the worst was behind us. We began to focus on the impact of the virus and the lockdown it had enforced. One image from that time still haunts me. It is the photograph of thirty-eight-year-old Ramrati, whom I reported on. A mother of three, she was rescued in a skeletal state—weighing just twenty-five kilos—by Rajni Gupta, Panipat's Women Protection and Child Marriage Prohibition Officer, and her team. Her husband had locked her inside a toilet in Rishpur village, Panipat. The space measured only three feet by three feet. She had been kept there for over a year. Stories like hers—of domestic violence and brutal isolation—were exacerbated by the lockdown.

A twelve-year-old girl had to save herself in UP's Bulandshahr from her own family who were marrying her off. Through her, I documented a dramatic shift in conversations around girls in rural communities. 'They will elope with lovers' was a common fear expressed by families with adolescent daughters during the interviews. Some poor families simply wanted to reduce the burden of feeding too many mouths, and so, the easiest solution was to marry off the girls. Many child marriages were attempted while the police machinery remained too overwhelmed to intervene.

While some stories like hers and Ramrati's were reported, there were many that remained confined in homes and villages.

Another rural storm rising was that of farmers marching to Delhi, challenging the three newly passed farm laws.

A nationwide vaccine drive was underway. There was a sense of ease among the masses. As a result, we let our guard down. Masks became accessories to be matched with our outfits. Christmas and New Year's Eve were celebrated with great gusto.

3

2021: The Dance of Death in Lucknow

The backstory of my coverage of the second wave was written in early April 2021. I was then a part of *ThePrint*'s political bureau headed by D.K. Singh. I was struggling to cover regional parties such as the SP, the BSP, the JJP for a while.

D.K. Singh asked me to do a profile of the Samajwadi Party patriarch, Mulayam Singh Yadav. He was hard to reach; Akhilesh Yadav was fiercely shielding his father from media glare. No party insider would divulge any details on how Netaji—as party workers affectionately addressed him—spent his days or what he thought of the current political scenario. The eighty-two-year-old former chief minister had ruled UP politics for decades, but a combination of poor health, the pandemic and the ascent of his son, all meant that the veteran was now confined to his home in Lucknow. Those close to the former CM told me that his health had worsened lately.

This would have been my breakthrough political byline ahead of the 2022 assembly elections in UP. I had to dig deeper and cultivate sources on the ground to flesh out my story. And so, I travelled to Lucknow.

As I stepped out of the plane at Lucknow airport on 8 April, I was stopped at a screening desk, which had two rules: either show a negative RT-PCR test or take a COVID test right there. Travel restrictions were in place, and everyone (including the crew and the passengers) had to wear a face shield and a mask. At the desk, I showed my negative report and moved on.

For the next two days, I explored the city, meeting various sources for the story, and mapping Lucknow's power corridors. When a friend wondered why I had not been to Madhurima Bakery yet, I jokingly said to Arunesh (my driver) that he wasn't taking me to the best restaurants.

On our way to the bakery, Arunesh, thirty-two, complained about the lockdown, the loss of jobs and the government's apathy towards the working class. He believed that government employees were getting their salaries as usual, while workers like him had no income. He believed the government owed the labour class some sort of financial aid.

When I told him that my trip would last for a week, he was relieved at the prospect of a week's work and drove me to the bakery, a wide smile on his face. 'You'd be surprised, madam, this is the first trip that I have got since last year,' he said. He had been doing odd jobs or simply sitting at home.

We reached the bakery in no time. There was a strange anxiety in the air. I ordered tea, and later some aloo-poori, but I could not eat breakfast.

I had no appetite. Perhaps I was disheartened at not getting through to Mulayam Singh Yadav. Though I had met Aparna Bisht Yadav, Mulayam Singh Yadav's stepson Prateek Yadav's wife, she hadn't spoken much. I had also visited the SP's office where they had asked me to deposit my phone at the reception and I had simply walked out in protest at this made-up rule. Later, I spent hours standing outside the residence of Mulayam Singh Yadav where I met a policeman who had been with him for the last decade. He tried to help, but there wasn't much he could do. My efforts to meet Akhilesh Yadav did not yield fruit, either—he had blocked my access to him because of an opinion piece published on our news portal. I tried to explain to a few of his team members that I wasn't the person who had written that piece, but they didn't budge.

Also, the pandemic was bearing down on me. In the past two-three days, I had seen some ambulances carrying dead bodies as I made my way back to my hotel.

On 10 April, I left my dinner uneaten. I wondered again if it was the sight of the ambulances or the continuous sound of the sirens that was making me anxious. On 11 April, I had nothing to do, my meetings were called off. I stepped out anyway. I could sense that everyone I met was on edge. Shopkeepers, cashiers at restaurants, drivers, passersby on the streets and I, we all shared a feeling of restless apprehension.

I checked the data. And that gave context to the sense of impending doom everywhere. Delhi Metro had shut various stations, COVID negative tests had become mandatory for air travel, and a license was required to keep restaurants open. Even the number of people gathering for seminars, workshops or lectures was restricted.

The number of active cases in Uttar Pradesh was astonishingly high. The number of new cases soared to a record high of 15,353 in a single day, with Lucknow bearing the brunt of the outbreak. The district accounted for 27 per cent of the total active cases, which surged from 3,912 on 1 April to 20,195 on 11 April—a staggering 500 per cent increase in just ten days.[1]

On the same day, a video of Lucknow's District Magistrate Abhishek Prakash talking to the doctors of a city hospital went viral. The Collector was saying, 'Increase ICU beds, put people in isolation, do whatever is possible as you people are experts … Because now, people are dying on the roads.' His voice quivered; it was echoing the city's terror. The situation was spiralling out of control.[2]

I set aside the Mulayam Singh Yadav profile and switched to COVID reporting. On 11 April, the roads were dominated by ambulances racing to hospitals or crematoriums. The vaccination centres now bore an abandoned look. The city soon became a ghost town, haunted by the spectre of the pandemic. It all happened within a week.

India had begun its COVID-19 vaccination drive on 16 January 2021, launching it in five initial phases. The rollout had begun with healthcare workers—nurses, doctors, paramedics—as the beneficiaries in Phase One. Phase Two, introduced two weeks later on 2 February, focused on frontline workers, including police personnel, sanitation staff, ambulance drivers and disaster responders.

In March, vaccinations were extended to senior citizens and individuals with comorbidities.

April widened the eligibility to all adults above forty-five, and by 1 May, the campaign was opened to every adult in the country, but by then vaccines had run out.

To get a clearer picture of the situation on the ground, I visited Baikunth Ghat, one of the largest cremation grounds in Lucknow, situated near the Gomti river, managed by Lucknow Nagar Nigam.

I saw families awaiting their turn for ten hours or more to cremate their loved ones. The ghat was working round the clock.

At the non-COVID queue, a dead body arrived every ten minutes. In the short time that I was there, I counted twenty-five bodies. There were two types of queues at the ghat. The COVID queue was designated for patients who had tested positive and were brought in from hospitals. The non-COVID queue, on the other hand, was for those who had passed away at home, en route to the hospital, at testing centres or due to sudden, unexplained causes.

There was no access to district administration except for the Municipal Commissioner, Ajay Dwivedi. From the sanitization of city lanes to creating new cremation grounds and bringing wood for pyres, the information he provided became the only verified intel available.

I dialled his number and requested a meeting. To my surprise, he agreed. No officer was willing to meet someone from the public at the time.

Dwivedi's wife was pregnant. He had isolated her and his parents at the government residence while he camped at his office.

Many public servants who were working during the second wave had isolated themselves from their families as they conducted public interactions. Those who were not able to isolate themselves refused to meet people.

Dwivedi looked exhausted. Every time somebody tweeted a photo of overburdened cremation grounds, it was him people held accountable because he was the only one responding from the Lucknow administration. If he didn't, it would not go down well with the government.

During our meeting, he called his subordinates to get the official data on COVID and non-COVID deaths. On that day alone, the bodies of sixty-nine people who had died of COVID had come to Lucknow's crematoriums. Crematoriums were at capacity and understaffed because its workers had gone to the Kumbh Mela in Uttarakhand; bodies kept piling up. The Mela turned into a superspreader.

The staff that remained in Lucknow were too scared to handle these bodies because of the massive surge in infections. To meet the demand at the crematoriums, the municipal commissioner outsourced last rites to a hundred new workers working in two shifts, day and night.

In one of his interviews, Dwivedi had told a Hindi daily that he was trying to ensure that there weren't long queues at cremation grounds. More wooden pyres were being arranged. This interview greatly upset the public. 'So they want more people to die? Shameful. Disgusting. The focus is not on arranging for oxygen cylinders and providing hospital beds but on building pyres to cremate the dead,' someone wrote on social media.

But his job was to ensure that there was no shortage of wood pyres and electric cremation facilities. Being a municipal commissioner, he could not have arranged beds at the hospital, that was the Collector's responsibility. By 13 April, within two days, the municipal commissioner had got fifty funeral pyres built by the newly sourced staff in the night, so there were fewer queues the next morning.

As the administration was busy employing new people, wood kept running out again and again. To meet this new demand, Dwivedi started getting wood from the adjoining district of Sitapur. Ten trucks were roped in to ferry wood to the cremation grounds in Lucknow. Since COVID-affected bodies were coming in unprecedented numbers, five new electric crematoriums were under construction in the third week of April. The old ones were overworked, and several machines stopped working. One electric crematorium could handle not more than eight-ten bodies in twenty-four hours.

I kept visiting both Gulala Ghat and Baikunth Ghat. The smell of burning flesh was nauseating. The situation on the ground was much worse than the state health bulletin showed. According to the state health bulletin of 12 April, seventy-two COVID patients had died in the preceding twenty-four hours in UP, of which twenty-one deaths happened in Lucknow. The corresponding figures in 13 April's bulletin for the preceding twenty-four hours were eighty-five for the state and eighteen for the city.[3]

Dozens of families were waiting for their turn to perform the last rites of their loved ones. At Gulala Ghat, thirty-three–year–old Ajay Kumar sat cluelessly—his uncle had succumbed to the virus.

'My mausa-ji was sick for a week. He complained of fever and cough, and died within one day of hospitalisation,' he said.

As families said their goodbyes to loved ones, ghat employees continued to prepare new pyres. Suresh, a young man in his late twenties, an employee at Gulala cremation ground, had broken his leg in an accident. But since there was too much to do at the cremation ground, he had no choice but to show up every day dragging his plastered leg along.

At the counter, distressed families pushed and shoved each other to get ahead and find out more about the process to cremate a COVID body.

Even Suresh was horrified, 'I have never seen a situation like this. I have seen more dead bodies in one week than in my whole life.'

The health machinery in the state capital was failing. To publish a full report on COVID-19 deaths, I had to get the hospital's version from the main COVID facility at King George's Medical University (KGMU).

There was a crowd outside the COVID ward. In the outer premises, families lay under the sun, waiting.

Three dead bodies were brought to the hospital just then, their families crying helplessly. I did not have the courage to go to them. I just stood there, captured an image on my phone and left. I called the numbers of the state health department's principal secretary, the chief medical officer of Lucknow, the district magistrate and other authorities who were responsible for COVID-19 management, but I didn't get a response. Their phones were ringing non-stop and most numbers were either busy or out of network coverage area.

Dr D.S. Negi, director-general of UP's health department eventually came on record to give some insights.

'This spike can be attributed to Holi when people come from all over the country to their hometowns. The general public's attitude towards the virus has become too casual.'

Another insider from the medical fraternity, Dr M.N. Siddiqi of Integral Medical College concurred.

'Even if you go to the market, 50 per cent of the people won't be wearing a mask. Healthcare workers are now getting infected in en masses. The second wave is more lethal as the jump in the proportion of infected patients worsening to critical illness has gone up to 50 per cent in comparison to the first wave,' he explained.

'Most of the government and private hospitals in the city are full. But now many of these hospitals are turning their isolation wards into ICUs to accommodate critical patients, as people from neighbouring districts are also coming to Lucknow,' Dr M.N. Siddiqi added.

I tried to meet the Collector via his office but there was no response, so I decided to head towards his residence. Security guards stopped us at the gate. One of them, with a cloth mask on his chin, walked towards our car and spoke through the car window.

'Sahab aur unki family ko jabse COVID hua hai tab se yahaan par toh sirf security guard hain.' (Since sir and his family have been infected with COVID, only us guards and staff have been here.)

Usually, guards at government residences shoo you away or have no interest in providing details about their boss, but this guard engaged me in a conversation. He proceeded to ask more questions about the situation. He was tense about his own test results. He had mistaken me as one of the members of the medical team. I clarified to him that I was a journalist covering the pandemic.

'Humari terah staff walon ki report nahin aayi hai madam. Bataa dete toh ghar par thoda savdhani barat lete.' (We haven't yet received the test reports of thirteen staff members. If they updated us about the result, we could warn our families to stay safe.)

The staff at this residence weren't provided N-95 masks. They were using their cloth masks. I had some extra N-95s, so I gave one to the security person talking to me and left.

Chief Minister Yogi Adityanath was reviewing the crisis through video conferences and ground inspection. After his visit on 11 April, he ordered the closure of all government and private schools and private coaching centres, till 30 April.[4] In the week that followed, the hospitals that had been sending COVID patients back—Lucknow's Era Medical College, T.S. Mishra Medical College and Integral Medical College—were also listed as COVID dedicated hospitals.

The state government announced that 2,000 ICU beds would be added in Lucknow by the next day, and another 2,000 in the next seven days. By 13 April, all of UP was put under a strict night curfew beginning at 9 p.m., after which only people with special passes were allowed to move about outdoors.[5]

The details of a city crumbling under the weight of the pandemic made it to my report published on 14 April. What followed this story became one of the most defining stories of coverage.

THE UNDERCOUNTING OF DEATHS

When I met Municipal Commissioner Ajay Dwivedi, he had shared the real time data on COVID and non-COVID deaths sourced directly from the city crematoriums. There was a huge gap between his statistics and the numbers on the health bulletin. There was more to this than met the eye.

I checked the health bulletin of 14 April.[6] It claimed that fourteen people had died of COVID in Lucknow. But Dwivedi's figures said otherwise: 101 cremations had taken place in the Hindu cremation grounds. The data from cremation grounds for Muslims and Christians wasn't even included in his update.

He left it to me to figure out the undercounting. And even though he shared with me the data he had access to, he refused to give an official statement. How was I going to make sense of these numbers?

My editor, D.K. Singh suggested, 'Go and count the dead bodies. The bodies won't lie.'

And that's how I took the lid off the big cover-up.

Following my report, a few news channels started broadcasting visuals suggesting that the actual number of deaths was being kept from the public. But how many were dying, what was the gap between real time figures and those on government portals?

At first, when D.K. Singh suggested I count the bodies, I had thought it too risky an idea. I would have to wear multiple layers of masks to prevent infection. Even then there was no guarantee that I wouldn't catch the virus. But I took the chance and spent the 14th and 15th of April at the ghats where Hindus were cremated. Uttar Pradesh reported 1,29,848 active cases on 15 April across the state. Lucknow continued to be the worst hit as the tally reached 35,865 active cases.[7]

At Mukti Dham, I met a staff member, twenty-nine–year–old Amar.

'Chaaro ore laashein hi laashein hai,' (There are dead bodies everywhere I look) he said, as we circumnavigated the burning pyres.

At six that evening, I saw thirty pyres burning at once, even as more bodies waited in queue to be consigned to flames. When I took out my phone to record the ghastly scene, I spotted four young men at a distance. They were stacking wood on one side of the ghat to prepare a row of funeral pyres for the next round of cremations.

When they saw me recording, they got nervous and started placing the wood here and there. I explained that I wasn't a government employee but a journalist. Relieved, they went back to work.

Among the dead bodies in the queue, one was of Manoj. I was told that he was in his late forties. He had complained of 'fever and body ache' before he died, a relative who stood there told me. 'We took him to every hospital that we could find in the city but no one admitted him.'

He didn't know whether Manoj was COVID positive or not. 'Jo zinda hain, unke test ka result to aa nahi raha, mare hue ka test kahaan se karaate.' (The test results of those who are alive are not coming on time, there is no question of the dead being tested.) Despite having had symptoms, Manoj was cremated in the section of the crematorium assigned to non-COVID bodies.

The cremation ground staff were not just overwhelmed, they were also underpaid and overworked. 'After Holi, the numbers started increasing. I haven't taken a holiday since last year. But just as I thought of taking one, sixty to sixty-five bodies started coming in every day,' a member of the staff at the Baikunth Dham crematorium told me. He said it wasn't just COVID, but the number of people dying otherwise too, had gone up.

There was no mechanism (or time) at the cremation grounds to identify who died of COVID and who died of TB or a heat stroke or cardiac arrest. This could be one reason why the government was underestimating the number COVID deaths. Only the bodies tagged by hospitals as having died of COVID were counted as COVID casualties. Rest, including those who were isolated at home or on the way to the hospital, or those who had remained untreated, never made it to the register of COVID deaths.

Some government insiders admitted that the collection of data was flawed. Some of the government officials I spoke to later in my assignment said that there was a 'lack of timely medical attention' at the peak of the crisis.

'Since not all of the people who died were tested, one can't say for sure whether those who were cremated at non-COVID funeral facilities weren't COVID positive,' a chief medical officer in eastern UP said to me. The World Health Organisation (WHO) estimated that more than 4.7 million people died due to COVID-19 in India. This figure was ten times higher than the number recorded by the Government of India. The Indian government rejected this figure claiming that the methodology adopted by WHO did not align with the state's records. Till date, the undercounting of COVID deaths remains a contentious issue because independent investigations do not match with official records.

When more and more videos from the Lucknow ghats started going viral, the municipal corporation officials decided to do something about it. The department deployed its lower and middle rank officers at the ground. The officials, in their sarkari vehicles with sirens on, started inspecting the ghats and its surrounding areas, checking the cremation queues and scolding the security guards at the ghats for sharing the number of dead bodies from the registers with the press.

To publish my story, I still needed the data for 13, 14 and 15 April from the cremation grounds, but the staff were restricted from speaking up.

The authorities went to the extent of covering the boundaries of Baikunth Dham with blue tin walls, preventing local photojournalists or the public from taking pictures.

So, I drove to the other side of the river, from where the burning pyres could be seen. I had barely stepped out of the car and pulled out my phone when I saw a Jeep coming towards me.

'Stop that! Filming this is strictly prohibited,' an official in plain clothes almost threatened me.

'Even media isn't allowed to cover?' I asked firmly. He asked me to leave. Arunesh and I left.

But I found a workaround.

Dyal Singh (name changed to protect his identity), the staffer at Mukti Dham, was an amiable person. He was in his late forties and quite articulate. He gave me his number and in the evenings, he started sending me voice notes about the number of COVID and non-COVID dead bodies. They came along with photos of the register's pages.

On 15 April, the Uttar Pradesh government's health bulletin recorded 104 COVID deaths in the last twenty-four hours.[8] Lucknow reported only twenty-six. However, what I gathered from the cremation grounds was quite different.

Till 6 a.m. on 15 April, Mukti Dham recorded twenty-eight COVID bodies and Baikunth Dham accounted for eighty. So, the tally for Lucknow was 108. On14 April, the government portal said that fourteen COVID bodies were cremated in Lucknow, but the number at both the ghats put together was 101. On 13 April, when eighty-four COVID bodies were cremated at both the ghats, the government data reflected merely eighteen deaths. The corresponding figures for 12 April at Mukti Dham and Baikunth Dham were ninety-two and twenty-one, respectively.

Now it was time for me to visit Lucknow's two major Christian cemeteries, and about a hundred big and small Muslim burial grounds to get an overall picture.

On the morning of 16 April, I decided to visit Aishbagh Kabristan, one of the biggest burial grounds in Lucknow. Here, too, people waited in a queue to bury their loved ones.

'We have registered over 350 bodies since 1 April, and the number has tripled since last month,' said a member of the managing committee responsible for operations at the burial ground.

'We didn't receive too many COVID bodies in February and March but have buried twenty-two such bodies since 1 April. But what's more alarming is the high number of "non-COVID bodies" that we have been getting in the last few days,' he added.

Once I was done reporting the story, I needed to get a comment from either additional chief secretary, Health and Family Welfare, Amit Mohan Prasad, or Lucknow Collector, Abhishek Prakash but it was nearly impossible. Ever since Abhishek Prakash's video about 'people dying on roads' had gone viral, he was lying low. The video was an admission from the government that people were, in fact, dying on roads. When he became inaccessible, the public anger got diverted towards the municipal commissioner, Ajay Dwivedi. Nagar Nigam was already running out of funds, claimed Dwivedi.

'On top of that, we have to spend eight-ten lakh rupees every day for pyre wood. We are ordering five quintals of wood every day,' he shared.

We published the story on 16 April with the headline, 'Reality of Lucknow's COVID Funerals Stands in Stark Contrast to UP Govt's Claims'.

4

A Death Live-Tweeted

I had been in Lucknow for more than a week, going from graveyard to graveyard. The city was racked with loss and grief.

It took a toll on me as well. Not just emotional but also physical.

My appetite was gone. Sickness crept in.

Until a week ago, Arunesh had been navigating the roads with a sceptic's mind. He would constantly bring up a conspiracy theory and we'd laugh about it.

'The government is planning something sinister. Maybe it wants to help hospitals and healthcare mafias by striking mortal fear of Corona in people. Corona vorona kuch nahin hai.' Corona is not a real thing. He would ask why it wasn't visible to the naked eye.

Each time he saw me emerging from the crematorium gates though, his conspiracy theory would fall apart. I would find him diligently sanitising his hands like me. My graveyard visits weighed heavily on him. As the days went by, he grew more and more concerned for his family. He was the lone breadearner in a family of half a dozen members who lived with limited means.

The April heat intensified the stress of reporting from a city ravaged by crisis. I was still struggling with food but found comfort in sipping coconut water. Arunesh offered khichdi and kaadha made by his mother; he told me her kaadha could bring back a dead man to life.

The simple taste of home actually made me feel a lot better.

As dawn broke on 17 April, Arunesh parked the car outside the hotel right on time. That morning, I had made up my mind to seek refuge in a different hotel, hoping that a change of place would help recover my appetite.

The new hotel room welcomed me with cheerful sunlight. It had a mango tree right outside the window. I always make it a point to choose rooms with sunlight and a window. The gloom of dim and shadowy rooms makes it very hard for me to write. All one needs is a desk by the window with natural light and a breeze. Over the years, this has become my way of coping with the solitude of travel and the strangeness of new places.

'Aaj phir shamshan?' Arunesh's voice cut through our routine as I got into the car after checking in. The word 'crematorium' hung between us like a spectre.

My mind was elsewhere that day. I was fixated on unravelling the knots of bureaucracy. That was the only way to understand the way the city was responding to the crisis.

'Take me to the city's COVID Command Centre in Lal Bagh,' I told Arunesh. I was looking for answers only the Chief Medical Officer (CMO) could have provided.

The COVID Command Centre was a fortress protected by barricades where a contingent of over two dozen policemen stood guard. A handful of media professionals stood ready with their camerapersons to chronicle these testing times.

By now, the city was a mosaic of queues—long lines at medical stores, weary processions at the COVID testing centres, anxious gatherings at hospitals and endless streams at the crematoriums. A queue had formed at the command centre.

The common thread that tied the queues together was sheer human desperation for one last chance at life.

Distressed family members clung to their phones—pleading with officials, their faces drenched in sweat and tears.

Some fought with the guards posted outside the gate, but their desperate efforts yielded no response from the men in uniform who were only trained to maintain order.

Others were so drained by the April sun that they took shelter under a tin shade, a tree or in the shadow of the barricades. Wives whose husbands were going to breathe their last any minute, were on the verge of losing consciousness. Young men and women cried helplessly.

Each sob was bound by only one hope: to secure a vital document from the CMO. This was no ordinary letter; it was the lifeline that would open the gates of hospitals for ailing patients. These families were turned away by the hospitals because they didn't possess this precious letter. The hospital officials expressed helplessness that they were only following the government's protocol.

These families were one letter away from saving the lives of their loved ones. Each moment counted.

Finally, the man arrived and the crowd rushed to the main gate of the centre. The CMO, however, avoided entering from the front gate where hopeful eyes awaited him.

I tried to request the policemen to allow me to meet him but to no avail. A few of them, torn between duty and empathy, looked away when I stared at them with disdain.

I decided to stand outside and wait for the CMO to emerge. On most days, Arunesh remained inside the car and waited for me to finish the task and return. But this time, he came out of the car to mingle with the distressed crowd. He talked to some of people and whispered about the 'journalist madam' he had been driving. It was there I met Harshit Srivastava. Unlike others, he stood vigil outside the office threshold. He was attending calls on one phone and replying to texts on another. Tears were running down his cheeks, and his hands were trembling.

Srivastava paused for a moment, cleaned his specs and started walking towards me. He had overheard Arunesh telling others that I was from the media.

His sixty-five-year-old father, Vinay Kumar Srivastava, a former journalist, needed urgent hospitalisation.

'His oxygen level has dropped,' he said, holding out his phone with a WhatsApp image that showed an SpO2 count of 50, much lower than the alarming 88.

His father needed critical care. A day before, he had complained of uneasiness, and by night, within a few hours, he was struggling to breathe.

Harshit went to three of Lucknow's prominent hospitals—Balrampur, Jagrani and Residency Era. Each one had refused to admit his father.

Harshit had found the CMO's office at Lal Bagh just this morning and he was determined to get the letter or he wouldn't return home.

By now his specs were fogged with tears; he could barely find the words to say more. Arunesh, who had been attentively listening to him, rushed to the car and returned with a water bottle.

'We ran from pillar to post but could not get an oxygen cylinder for him,' Harshit said. 'A relative lent us his own cylinder. I went to get it refilled at midnight but there was a long queue for that too. I had to fight the others to save my father,' with this, he started weeping again.

He had already had his father's COVID sample collected the morning before but the RT-PCR test results were not due for another three days. In the meantime, his father's health continued to deteriorate.

Of course, the long delay in test results cast a shadow of despair, but having to procure the CMO's letter had started to break his spirit altogether. It didn't matter that his father very obviously had symptoms of COVID.

CMO Sanjay Bhatnagar walked past us again. We tried to call out, but our voices simply dissipated in the air.

It was in this moment of helplessness that I decided to do something.

'Why not broadcast the severity of your father's condition on Twitter?' I asked Harshit and he gave his consent.

And so, one tweet at a time, we started chronicling his father's deteriorating health and oxygen levels.

It was a desperate measure, a digital cry for help. When his father's limited following didn't help,

I used my account. Within minutes of my retweeting, word spread far and wide.

The story resonated with a large number of people.

We tagged Shalabh Mani Tripathi, the then media advisor to Chief Minister Yogi Adityanath. His handle commanded influence and power, and he was using it actively respond to many SOS tweets. I mobilised every contact in my list.

Meanwhile, Harshit's wife called, asking him to return.

I offered him reassurance that I would scour the hospitals for a bed. We exchanged numbers.

'Keep your eyes on Twitter,' I urged him. 'The CM's office might reach out.'

Then I set out alone to find a hospital bed. As I navigated the city's COVID hospitals one after another, the story I witnessed remained uniform. St. Joseph, Sahara, Vivekanand, Mayo, Chandan and Balrampur hospitals—all turned me away by citing protocol. They wanted the CMO's letter.

Dozens of patients were denied admission as their family members raced against time in search of hospital beds while they languished in the backseats of cars or in the back of ambulances.

A COVID positive report meant nothing.

Every time, I confronted a hospital official about this, I got the same reply. The referral policy put in place by the state government was strictly being followed.

Now the battle was not just against the virus but against the very system designed to protect citizens.

On investigation, I found an official paper dated April 2020 and signed by the Collector.

'The decision related to hospital admissions will be taken by Dr Sanjay Bhatnagar, CMO, and the decision will be final,' the letter read.

This letter held more than procedural weight, it was the barrier between patients and the medical care they desperately needed.

After all my calls to Sanjay Bhatnagar went unanswered, I phoned another senior health department official. He didn't want to go on record but he offered a justification for the year-old directive.

'The decision was taken to regulate and keep an eye on COVID management,' he said. 'Without it, hospitals operate unchecked and make data tracking difficult for us.'

The CMO's referral letter, became representative of the bureaucracy's complexity and inefficiency when swift action was needed the most. One could argue that the bureaucracy was overwhelmed by an unprecedented crisis. But it was impossible to ignore the glaring oversight—the inability to anticipate the magnitude of this type of emergency was not just a procedural failure, but a tragic misstep with dire consequences.

Families like Harshit Srivastava's paid heavily for this. The end of a queue at a hospital's testing centre was the only point of entry for common citizens. Yet, they could get tested, yet there was no guarantee of admission.

At 3.35 p.m., I got a WhatsApp message that said—'My father is no more.'

This wasn't just another story in my journalistic pursuit, I had got personally involved to help a family, setting my work and health aside. I had never met Vinay Srivastava but it felt like a personal loss at the time.

I got back to the car, sat in silence for some time and then gathered the strength to respond, 'I am sorry for your loss.'

The last few days had affected Arunesh too. He witnessed what I saw, reported and wrote about. Now, he worried a lot more, and didn't laugh often enough.

Harshit's live tweets about his father's low oxygen levels and ultimately his death garnered attention but not action.

Shalabh Mani Tripathi's promise on Twitter that help was on its way meant nothing; no state official contacted Harshit to offer support. Google Maps led me to the barricaded entrance of Sector 12 in Vikas Nagar near Aliganj. In Harshit's neighbourhood, the guards refused to let outsiders in. It took thirty long minutes to persuade them that I was a relative and his father had just died.

Their lane was deserted. From a distance, we could hear people crying. Some people peeked through their balconies but were too afraid to come out and offer condolences to the grieving family.

I was about to step into a home where the virus had just claimed a life. The risk of contagion was high.

Harshit guided me to a room where the body draped in a sheet lay still on the bed.

Harshit's wife, Nishu, and mother, Aruna, were huddled around his father's body. The remnants of a lost battle surrounded them—Coronil, an oxygen cylinder and scattered strips of medicines.

His father had watched an ad on television which claimed that Coronil could save lives but the virus claimed him before he could even commence his treatment.

Beyond this personal tragedy, there was a larger story, waiting to unfold in the coming years.

In June 2020, just three months after India recorded its first COVID case, Baba Ramdev announced that he had found a cure. His company, Patanjali Ayurved, launched a pill called Coronil which would cure the virus within seven days of infection.[1]

The controversial medicine, heavily criticised for its unscientific claim, fed into the desperation of millions seeking a cure. In fact, it became so popular that the company sold 25 lakh Coronil kits within four months of its launch, earning 250 crores.[2] These numbers are astonishing despite the fact that the AYUSH Ministry (Ayurveda, Yoga & Naturopathy, Unani, Siddha & Homoeopathy) had banned Patanjali from selling the pills, after which Patanjali rebranded it as an 'immunity booster'.[3]

Front page ads and a high profile launch on 19 February 2021 helped Patanjali record a sharp increase in sales during the second wave.[4]

Two cabinet ministers—Dr Harsh Vardhan, Health Minister, and Nitin Gadkari, the Minister for Road Transport and Highways—attended the event where Baba Ramdev repeated his claim of curing and preventing COVID-19 with Coronil, attracting widespread criticism from India's medical fraternity.[5] The presence of India's health minister was criticised by the largest doctors' body, IMA (Indian Medical Association).[6]

Three years later, for misleading advertisements and claims, Patanjali faced scrutiny from the Supreme Court of India.

In early 2024, a bench comprising Justice Hima Kohli and Justice A. Amanullah summoned Baba Ramdev and Acharya Balkrishna to court in person and directed them to publish an unconditional apology. When the duo appeared in court to personally apologise, the court rejected the apology.[7]

The bench used strong remarks such as 'the country is being taken for a ride', 'will rip you apart' and also criticised the state for 'sitting with its eyes shut'.

The verdict of the case came in August 2024. Eventually, the Supreme Court closed the contempt case against Ramdev and Balkrishna, accepting their apologies, but not without a strict warning. They were cautioned against any future violation of court orders.[8]

In the room where Harshit's father lay, his family expressed regret at being unable to offer me even the simplest hospitality of tea or water. The weight of their apology sat heavy on my heart..

The pandemic had isolated the family in their grief. Not a single neighbour came forward to offer help or condolences.

Harshit lamented to the silent figure, who had once been his father, 'For thirty years, you championed journalism, extended a helping hand to all, and devoted your life's savings to COVID relief efforts. Now, in our hour of need, where is everybody?'

Some people on Twitter questioned which party Vinay Srivastava had voted for so that the crowd could decide whether to mourn or mock him.

Harshit tweeted, 'I voted for the nation.'

For the next half an hour, I sat between the bedroom and the living room as a silent witness.

In his last moments, Vinay had asked for food and the family had gathered around him for a meal.

The confirmation of Vinay's RT-PCR test arrived four days later. It was too late. The positive result was just a postscript to a lost life.

My report on Uttar Pradesh's COVID crisis and draconian referral letter, published by *ThePrint*, captured the world's attention, spurring the Yogi administration into action. Many national and international media houses followed up on Srivastava family's ordeal.[9]

In a decisive move, the government mandated that both private and public hospitals would admit not only those with confirmed RT-PCR positive results but also those who were suspected to be infected.

This directive came in the wake of an alarming trend—the RT-PCR results of patients with classic symptoms of COVID were turning out to be negative. The government acknowledged the reality that the virus could escape detection and still wreak havoc. Changes were made in the inclusion criteria for hospital admission, extending them to clinical diagnoses based on X-rays, CT scans and blood reports.

Harshit was once a devoted voter of the BJP. After the second wave, he found himself at a crossroads. He vowed to never vote for it. The schism spread through his family. He started getting into arguments with relatives who supported both CM Yogi and PM Modi.

'People's memories are short. They tend to believe whatever is shown on television. Despite the devastating loss my family and I endured, they vehemently deny the state's mishandling of the pandemic,' he shared with me during an interview in the midst of the 2024 Lok Sabha elections.

'When I state facts, their retort is simplistic: if not Modi and Yogi, then are we to vote for Muslims?' He highlighted the polarisation that drives elections in today's India.

Harshit also drew attention to the unchanged state of healthcare, 'Should COVID resurface, the history of mismanagement will be repeated because the health infrastructure has not progressed that much.'

Life has altered irrevocably for the Srivastava family. Their bitterness and cynicism are directed not only at the state's failure but also at close relatives who turned their backs on them.

'It was no ordinary death.' Harshit has saved the slip from the crematorium which affirmed his father's COVID-positive status, along with the test results from a lab. But the municipal corporation had denied a COVID death certificate to his father.

'My father remains excluded from the COVID statistics, despite testing positive.'

What counted as a COVID death, and what fell outside the official count? Not all who tested positive succumbed to the virus, not all who passed away were tested, and many who died in home isolation were never accounted for.

The absence of a unified global database also hampers policymakers', researchers' and even nations' assessment of the pandemic's magnitude.

In India, the question transcends policy. It probes the very heart of electoral democracy. Uttar Pradesh, one of India's most populous states, faced assembly polls in 2022, just a year after mass graveyards were photographed by media on the banks of the Ganges.

Journalists who reported from the state sought answers to the most pressing question: 'Will the large number of cremations and the lack of oxygen and hospital beds lead to the fall of Yogi Adityanath's government?'

It did not. Yogi Adityanath was elected for a second term. Mismanagement of the COVID crisis wasn't a poll issue. Even the constituencies which bore the brunt of the pandemic's fury voted for the BJP.

As the country moved closer to its eighteenth Lok Sabha elections in 2024, the opposition's campaigns barely touched upon the Modi government's handling of the pandemic. Despite being the most devastating health crisis since India's independence, COVID-19 failed to emerge as a defining poll issue in the 2024 general elections. A crisis that took lives, disrupted the nation's economy and upended the very idea of good governance was brushed aside, and got lost in the noise of other political narratives.

Instead, it is Narendra Modi who stuck to his narrative of resilience and reform during the trying times. In an interview to ANI's Smita Prakash, he claimed that his decade minus the two COVID years at the helm had yielded more progress in the country than the preceding seventy years of Congress rule.[10]

The BJP strategically added Modi's COVID management to their 2024 manifesto.[11] The party's narrative being the Modi government's handling surpassed even developed nations such as America which struggled with mass casualty during the virus outbreak.

There were several explanations to why the poor handling of a pandemic didn't lead to widespread dissent among the electorate.

Firstly, the political messaging which paints the Modi government's efforts as a triumph over the virus has resonated with its loyal voter base.

Secondly, TV news continues to capture the nation's imagination. What is broadcast on television is often considered gospel truth. The difference between TV coverage and the more critical reports from digital and print media meant that the latter's ground-level exposes failed to bring about any significant change in opinions.

Thirdly, COVID remains in the collective memory as just a tapestry of stories, not a catalogue of grievances against the state.

My travels through rural and small-town India in the following years revealed a pattern. People spoke of divine interventions during the pandemic rather than systemic failure. Women spoke of planning second and third pregnancies driven by pandemic fears.

Some recounted lessons in discipline learnt by standing in queues. Some boasted of their rural lifestyle, immunity and family genes during the virus outbreak.

Amidst these stories, voices that directly challenge the state or its legislators are very few. This silence tells us a lot about the complex interplay of memory, media and the machinery of governance.

5

Overburdened Smaller Towns

As Lucknow ran out of hospital beds, patients began to flock to the neighbouring districts of Barabanki and Sitapur. Families drove miles with their dying relatives cramped in the back seats of vehicles with life support from oxygen cylinders.

They weren't met with open arms and vacant hospital beds.

The rural districts' medical infrastructure was already stretched beyond its limits.

I travelled to Sitapur and Barabanki districts on 18 and 19 April. The state capitals and metro cities across the nation had buckled under the crisis, and the struggle of tier two and tier three towns remained unacknowledged by the national media.

As I journeyed through districts towns, the scenes unfolding before me starkly contradicted what the health bulletins said.

The police were deployed at oxygen plants. Hospitals gasping for breath had no choice but to deny new admissions. At Barabanki's Mayo Hospital, I saw a member of staff catching a moment of rest at the reception in between day and night shifts, the exhaustion writ large on his face.

Today, the idea of police guarding oxygen plants sounds stranger than fiction. But it was a reality back then. We will discuss the reasons behind the Indian state taking such extraordinary measures later in the chapter.

Much like the rest of the country, the number of cases in UP kept climbing. According to the state health bulletin, the number of active cases reached 2,23,544 on 20 April, with 163 deaths in twenty-four hours. Sitapur and Barabanki reported 219 and 347 fresh COVID cases, respectively, on 20 April.[1]

In truth, the numbers were higher. Many people went untested for various reasons—different for different segments of society. For instance, Mayo Hospital had made a conscious decision to not test its doctors, nurses and other medical staff. An administrator said to me off the record that testing was avoided as it might have shown that many of the frontline workers were themselves COVID-positive. All hands were required to be on the deck, every single staff member was indispensable, such was the scale of the pandemic. So, from sweepers to ward boys, from security guards to the nurses and doctors, all worked round the clock.

Here, I met Dr Bilal. He had practised maintaining a professional detachment in the face of loss, he said to me as we talked through a glass window while he stood inside the COVID ward and I remained outside. He was cautious about not wanting to pass on the virus in case he was a carrier.

What he had witnessed in the past week had broken him. For the first time in his professional life, he had cried. The more he talked about the situation, the more he struggled to finish his sentences.

We don't witness our doctors' shattered spirits every day.

'See, I can't hold back my tears. I feel helpless seeing the devastation …' I had stopped chasing after powerful, dramatic quotes for my stories by now—his tears spoke more than words could ever convey.

Policemen deployed at various hotspots were especially vulnerable, so they chose to remain untested. Many district officials too had fallen sick. A senior official from Barabanki, on the condition of anonymity, said, 'The morale has hit rock bottom. Just last week, the person who used to sit next to my office, succumbed to the virus. This fortnight, we have mourned five officials who worked at the block level. When we got them tested, we found that many BDOs (Block Development Officials) and Lekhpals were also infected.' He highlighted that 25 per cent of the district administration workforce was grappling with the infection.

Three family members of the officer were also COVID-19 positive. One of his senior colleagues' wife, pregnant with their second child, had been infected along with their firstborn.

It was worse for officers who were posted in the field at block, sub-division and district levels as their job involved not just attending VCs but also public meetings and COVID inspections.

The UP panchayat polls loomed large amidst this firefighting, tragically diverting the focus and resources of the state from the health crisis.

'The panchayat polls are upon us. Despite everything, we have to ensure that they also remain a priority,' the officer quoted above said. UP was simply walking into a catastrophe.

While the pandemic worsened, panchayat elections consumed most of the administrative officials' time and energy.

They had little say in this decision.

'The scheduling of the polls is not within our purview. Our duty lies solely in the execution,' the Barabanki official clarified. This sentiment was echoed by many officers in various districts as I travelled deeper into the state.

The electoral pursuit of the state government killed more than 2,000 educators. Government school teachers put on election duty paid a heavy price for this.

Rahul Khare, thirty, had driven from Lucknow to Mayo Hospital with his uncle (sixty-two) and cousin (thirty-one), both of whom were gasping for breath. The hospital had already plastered notices at its gates that said in bold letters, 'NO ICU BEDS AVAILABLE'.

Khare explained the patients' condition to the staff at the reception. 'His SpO2 is 91,' he said of his uncle, his voice calm but loaded with fear, 'And my cousin's is 85.'

The hospital staff had to turn away both patients. They had run out of beds for Level 2 and Level 3 patients. Khare's uncle and cousin were Level 2—they required oxygen support but were not yet critical enough to be put on ventilators.

Patients were categorised based on the severity of their condition. Level 1 patients could be treated in isolation at home. Level 3 required ventilators. Level 2, like Khare's relatives, needed a constant flow of oxygen supply along with vigilant medical care.

During the second wave, the condition of Level 2 patients was deteriorating to Level 3 within hours. That was what had happened to Harshit Srivastava's father.

Oxygen cylinders were a lifeline that many families were able to secure. Some families even managed to get multiple cylinders. But the reality was that this lifeline was a mere stopgap. Yet people began to hoard cylinders and private vendors began to sell them at jacked-up prices.We saw profiteering in its most brutal form. Oxygen cylinders, already in short supply, were being sold at exorbitant prices. When private vendors exhausted their stock, desperate families turned to oxygen plants on the outskirts of cities. But instead of aid, they were met with uniformed officers and barricades, their pleas drowned out by the state..

Rahul Khare also arranged two cylinders for his uncle and cousin from a local plant in Lucknow, but they needed a hospital to shelter them.

As Khare tried to plead with the hospital staff, I stood at a distance. Soon, I offered to listen to his plight.

'In Lucknow, I heard that patients are getting admitted to hospitals in neighbouring districts, where beds are still available.'

Beside the reception, under the shadow of a poster declaring 'No More Beds', a staffer who had succumbed to exhaustion, woke up.

He said that he had not been able to sleep for the last three days from fatigue.

'My legs have become numb. I feel nothing,' he pointed towards his swollen feet.

Right then, a speeding car made its way to the hospital reception. Another COVID patient and their distressed family came out.

Some men got out of the car; the patient, masked and tethered to an oxygen cylinder, remained in the backseat. Khare watched the men from a distance only to hear the harrowing refrain—no bed available.

That patient breathed his last in front of all of us.

Having made frantic calls to distant relatives for help and receiving none, Khare left, crestfallen.

After a while, I also left Mayo Hospital to visit the district hospital and the primary health centre in the district.

Surprisingly, there were long queues for testing.

The stigma around the virus and the fear of the unknown deterred citizens from getting tested during the first wave. The second wave had flipped the situation.

Now, awareness spread as promptly as the virus did; the sheer number of deaths had become impossible to ignore. Communities that once hesitated to get tested now showed paranoia. People understood that the knowledge of detection was the only weapon against the virus.

When I visited two COVID testing centres in Sitapur and Barabanki, at least fifty people were queued up at the Sitapur testing centre and more than sixty at Barabanki. Most people I interviewed complained of fever, cough and body ache.

Despite willingness among citizens, the district administrations had to enforce a limit on the daily collection of COVID-19 samples to prevent the flood of test samples from overwhelming the laboratories in Lucknow. This caused frustration among those who stood in long queues to get tested.

The assistant district health officer in Sitapur district, P.K. Singh, told me that the cap on daily RT-PCR tests was a 1,000 samples. Previously, it was limited to 800 samples.

'The worst affected districts are allowed to increase the number of samples dispatched to Lucknow,' he added.

The load bearing down on Lucknow's labs was evident from the interviews of numerous patients who lamented that it took up to or over seven days to receive test results.

Remember how the medical staff were not being tested?

On one hand, many frontline workers refrained from testing for the virus. Their rationale was one of sacrifice. The system was stretched to its limit and could not afford to part with any help they had.

On the other hand, there were students, housewives and the elderly, who had been confined to their homes for months and were now coming out to form these long testing lines.

In Barabanki, the strain was greater than in Sitapur. The day I reached, they were dispatching 971 RT-PCR tests, 1,263 antigen tests and 5 TrueNat tests to Lucknow, each test a different method of virus detection.

As I journeyed in the district, I found a COVID help desk at the railway station in Barabanki, designed to offer travellers the latest information about the virus and to screen them for infection. COVID help desks were found at many public transit points such as railway stations and bus stands during the second wave.

But the desk at Barabanki station lay deserted. It could be either due to understaffing or unpreparedness on the part of officials. A large number of pilgrims were returning to North Indian states from the superspreader event that the Kumbh Mela in Uttarakhand had turned out to be. So, the absence of officials was alarming because their deployment at COVID help desks could have been key to blocking the virus before it infiltrated villages.

At a bus stop in Sitapur, I met five men who had arrived from the Mela. They waited at the help desk for some time before heading towards their hometowns—without being screened.

Away from this chaos in smaller towns, the situation in the capital was getting worse every day. Within a week of the crisis, the situation spiralled beyond the control of the state and the central governments.

New Delhi, being one of the most affected cities, got into a tug-of-war with neighbouring states, accusing them of not letting oxygen carriers reach its hospitals. Delhi's hospitals were on the brink of collapse as thousands of patients were running out of oxygen supply. The Delhi government started to broadcast this on social media platforms with urgent pleas for help. Soon, this was reduced to theatrics.

The judiciary had to step in as the central government stood in silence, watching the battle play out between Delhi and other states the Delhi High Court reprimanded the central government, 'Beg, borrow, steal, it's your job to get oxygen.'[2]

The Indian Express reported that the Court's directive came on the heels of pleas by the Max Healthcare network. The hospital had sought urgent intervention as most of its hospitals were working with 'dangerously low levels of oxygen supply.'

The High Court then delivered a harsh critique of the Modi administration, 'We are shocked and dismayed that the government does not seem to be seeing the reality … What is happening? Human lives are not that important for the state.'

Beyond the scrutiny of courts, in the quiet corners of smaller towns, the oxygen plants stood under siege by the state and by desperate citizens. The police guarded them day and night. To make sense of the situation, I reached out to a doctor from Barabanki's Hind Hospital. He advocated for Z-level security at oxygen plants and ancillary medical facilities.

'People have become so desperate to claw back a fading pulse that they are not just attacking doctors but also the oxygen plants.' He narrated the harrowing episodes of violence against medical staffers.

Lately, his dreams consisted of someone's oxygen level falling to 50, or some attendant charging at him for failing to save their loved ones or of people with folded hands, begging for an oxygen cylinder.

The situation at Hind Hospital had grown so dire that the district administration had to deploy a Naib Tehsildar at the nearby oxygen plant along with the police force. A sub-divisional magistrate (SDM) was also assigned to the hospital as an overseer to protect the precious oxygen supply.

The hospital was designed to accommodate 340 patients in general, but had only 140 beds that were connected to oxygen. It was operating on less than half its capacity, and even for the 140 beds, oxygen supply dwindled with each passing moment.

At Mayo Hospital, the total number of oxygen-supported beds was supposed to be 260 but the hospital couldn't promise a sustained supply for much longer.

The situation was no different in Sitapur. I interviewed a health official overseeing the distribution of oxygen. 'Every COVID patient is watched by a family attendant. The attendants have become the custodians of oxygen cylinders. They fear that the moment a cylinder is left unattended, someone might steal it.'

The police were summoned to watch over the COVID ward, to prevent attendants from stealing oxygen cylinders from other patients.

'Despite the police watching over the COVID ward, no one is listening to the administration,' the official complained.

I decided to go back to Lucknow. Just when we were exiting the city, two young men on a scooty started swearing at Arunesh, and banging on my car window.

The more I requested Arunesh to ignore the men's provocations and focus on reaching the hotel on time, the more aggressive the two men got. I desperately wanted to avoid confrontation. When Arunesh braked, I hoped the men would move on, but they turned around once more and came closer. I pointed my phone camera at them to show I was recording their actions.

All of a sudden, the man riding pillion, lunged forward to grab my phone.

'Zyada video banaani aati hai madam ko?' (Madam likes making videos, huh?) he sneered at me.

I snatched my phone back but ended up bruising my hand. The duo then started their scooty and left.

Two men harassed a woman on the road and got away with it. I was shocked but in that moment I resolved to bring them to justice. If they got away without any consequences, they would do this again and again. Their misguided bravado needed to be checked.

I gathered my wits and urged Arunesh to pursue the scooty. I wanted to note down its number in order to register my complaint with the police. But the scooty did not have a number plate.

In response to our pursuit, they mocked us by flashing their phones, booing at me as they zig-zagged dangerously on the road. During this chase, I spotted traffic police at a chauraha and I asked Arunesh to stop and seek their intervention.

One of the traffic policemen asked us to seek help from a police vehicle that could be patrolling nearby. We crossed some distance and found a patrolling vehicle parked under a tree. I hurried over to the policemen, who were busy watching something on their phones and I recounted the incident.

The policemen acted swiftly, following us as we resumed our chase. Within a few minutes, we managed to overtake and stop the two men. Unaware of the cops behind us, they started to walk up to me, when one of the policemen rushed to grab the collar of one of them who was now aggressively hurling abuses at me. I was about to break down but somehow put on a brave face.

I called up, Yamuna Prasad, the superintendent of police (SP) of Barabanki. He assured me that action would be taken. He then spoke to one of the policemen who had rounded up the men and directed him to take us to the nearest police station.

On our way to the police station, I started having second thoughts. This was one of the few instances when I had decided not to brush the matter under the carpet. I asked myself if I was taking it too far, pursuing this case when I should have rushed back to the hotel to file my reports. This wasn't my first time travelling solo as a reporter. Harassment, being constantly mansplained to, casteism, sexism, etc., are all routine experiences. But this time, enough was enough.

The police station looked like any other moffusil police stations you find across small-town India. Its jurisdiction included the outskirts of the city where the incident had happened. One half of its force was scattered across town, in the COVID hotspots, and the other half was present in the station.

The SHO (station house officer) was sitting at a desk in the verandah to get some air, surrounded by a few juniors.

I sat across the SHO's desk and narrated the episode for the third time. He didn't seem to be in a hurry.

The scooty men, loosely handcuffed to one of the policemen, kept trying to approach the SHO, blabbering on about how Arunesh had deliberately hit them so they had lost a slipper. This offended a female officer, and she reprimanded them in a loud voice, 'You dare to harass a woman and then show such brazenness before the SHO?'

The SHO remained unfazed.

The men then started to address me, pleading for leniency.

'Where are your masks? You are riding a scooty without a number plate?' The female officer snapped at them again.

The SHO was impervious to the urgency, so I had no option but to reach out to Yamuna Prasad again. And all of a sudden, the policemen's grip on the men tightened, and my complaint was registered.

The scooty men started whispering urgently into their phones, calling their kin to rally for them in Lucknow. They weren't from Barabanki, they had been driving down from Lucknow.

They mention the impending legal outcomes of the complaint: 'Mahila waala case karaa dengi. Court le jayengi.' (She will file charges of harassment and drag us to court.)

I could sense fear in their tone now. They knew that I had digital evidence on my phone. I showed the footage to the SHO so he could allow me to write down my complaint.

I was given a pen and paper. The SHO instructed me to write in 'proper Hindi'. Each word I wrote in the complaint was met with resistance from the SHO. His interruptions were meant to discourage a woman who had been harassed from filing a complaint.

'Gaon ka address deejiye, Dilli ka nahi chalega, pitaji ka bhi address.' (Your village address, not your Delhi address. Add your father's too), he insisted when I wrote down the temporary address of my rented home in Delhi.

He called in Arunesh and prodded him to disclose the whereabouts of villages, making him nervous.

'Sir hum toh Lucknow mein rehte hain. Pitaji kabhi rehte the gaon mein, hum toh kabhi gaye nahin. Koi zameen bhi nahin hai. Pitaji khud nahi jaate udhar,' Arunesh told the SHO. (Sir, I live in Lucknow. My father used to live in the village. I have never set foot there. We have no land there. Nobody from my family lives there anymore.)

When I finished writing the report, the SHO walked me to the gate. 'Look, madam, they are both drunk. They've come from Lucknow amidst the lockdown to roam around and have fun. You're an educated woman from Delhi. It's better to hush this incident.'

He told me not to push for an FIR because fighting the case in a local court would be an inconvenience. He said that he was just asking me to be practical. The price, he said, would be paid by me in loss of money, time and most importantly, peace of mind.

He waved over the scooty men.

'Madam, we are sorry. We vow never to repeat such behaviour with any woman in the future.'

I shouldn't have had to face their abuse in the first place but I chose to let it go, hoping they had learnt their lesson.

I left for Lucknow, which was twenty-four km away.

6

A Breathless City

I collapsed as soon as I entered my hotel room that evening. Everything hurt. I had a sore throat, a fever and chest pain. All signs pointed to COVID. Again. It wasn't surprising considering I was going to all the places others were mortally afraid of. The first infection didn't immunise against the second variant. It was being said that the Delta variant was highly transmissible and way more dangerous; people as young as me were succumbing to the virus. Everyone was at risk. Journalists were conspicuously absent from the government's list of frontline workers, and therefore, not prioritised for vaccination.

As the night stretched on, my mind was in turmoil. I called up a senior colleague in Delhi.

'Get yourself tested and if it's COVID, rest. Get some rest even if it's not,' she said.

The more I thought about contracting COVID again, the more breathless I became. I didn't have an oximeter. I had medicines for fever, headache and ORS packets, but nothing to soothe my throat. My body had been weakened by weeks of skipped meals, lost appetite and dehydration. My legs trembled as I walked around the room. I spoke to Sangeeta in Delhi to arrange for a COVID test and an oximeter. But she couldn't.

In desperation, I dialled the laboratories in the city for an urgent test. Each call was met with, 'perhaps tomorrow or the day after'. Some said there was a three-day queue for sample collection.

I turned to Arunesh. To my utter shock, he, who earlier believed the pandemic to be a scam, had got himself vaccinated.

He drove me to hospitals that were conducting tests. I gave my sample at one where the waiting time was relatively short and on my way back, went to various pharmacies for an oximeter. The scarcity of this basic medical equipment was devastating. People were willing to pay 5,000 rupees for an oximeter, which cost anywhere between 500 to 1500 rupees. Even generic medicines such as paracetamol were in short supply. After running around for a while, I returned to the hotel, exhausted and without an oximeter.

Arunesh resumed the search without me. A while later, he sent me a picture of a steamer priced at 700 rupees, three times its actual price.

Meanwhile, my colleague Moushumi Das Gupta, who had also come to Lucknow, connected me with a doctor she knew, who prescribed the necessary medicine and asked me to take steam.

Arunesh brought food from his home. The food and steam felt like a balm. The next day, I found an oximeter for 2,500 rupees. For the next few days, I remained isolated in my room. The hotel staff would deposit food outside my door.

I needed to expedite my test result. With the help of a friend who was acquainted with a hospital's owner, I got my test result earlier than expected. Fortunately, it was negative. But the symptoms lingered.

As April neared its end, not just Lucknow's but the entire country's crematoriums became the epicentre for media houses. News outlets such as *Reuters*, the *BBC* and *CNN* started broadcasting haunting images of funeral pyres. Flames from cities such as Bhopal, Delhi, Surat, Ranchi, Mumbai, Lucknow and Varanasi engulfed screens around the world.

In Lucknow, even as the infected reporters were confined to their homes, they kept filing stories, relying on their sources and photographer colleagues who provided photos and videos from the ground.

A photograph of me exiting Baikunth Dham had also made it to the front page of a prominent Hindi daily in Uttar Pradesh, eliciting concern but also excitement from friends and readers.

With a negative report in hand, I stepped out once again to chase a story. Around that time, it was estimated that more than 5,000 patients were isolated in their homes in Lucknow city alone. Their families were managing symptoms through telephonic consultations, or going by whatever they read online. For some patients, each breath was dependent on an oxygen cylinder or concentrator.

After the Yogi government withdrew the CMO reference letter rule,[1] it issued an order on 21 April prohibiting the supply of oxygen to individuals and reserving it exclusively for hospitals, thus making the state the custodian of oxygen.

These orders precipitated an emergency-like situation on the ground. On the afternoon of 22 April, Zafar Abbas, forty-four, was arrested by Lucknow police as he was tending to a newly refilled oxygen cylinder.

Abbas was a resident of Kazmain Road in Turiya Ganj. He urgently required an oxygen cylinder for his father, eighty-five-year-old, Shahryar Hussain. Abbas was locked up at Sahadatganj police station for seven hours.

He told me on the phone that 'The police arrested me around 3.30 p.m. and didn't release me until about 11.00 p.m.' He lost not only the cylinder but also precious hours crucial for his father's treatment.

'Oxygen cylinders will be given to those who have a doctor's prescription. Without it, no oxygen cylinder shall be sold or distributed. This is to puncture the black market of oxygen supply,' a source in the government told me. To understand this chaos firsthand, I visited the main gas manufacturing sites in the city, where I saw long queues of people waving letters from doctors and public hospitals at the police force to be allowed to refill their cylinders. They were met with apathy.

The government's mandate to only allow hospitals to monitor oxygen clearly brought countless COVID patients isolated in their homes to harm.

Outside the Murari Gas Station in Nadarganj, some desperate family members fought with the police, while some made heartwrenching appeals. The cops, too, were helpless; their own families were battling the virus.

This plant had been supplying oxygen for free to those in need until the government passed the order.

A stone's throw away from Murari Gas Station stood Shrinathji Gases, where another squad of uniformed officers turned away desperate families pleading for oxygen. According to a *BBC* report, about 500 factories across India supplied liquid oxygen distilled from air at an extremely low temperature, often sourced from cryogenic plants, to hospitals through cylinders and tankers.

These scenes of anguish played out at every oxygen station. Shrinathji and Murari Gas Station were the sole providers of oxygen to Lucknow's hospitals—Shrinathji supplied to Lok Bandhu and Balrampur hospitals, Murari sustained forty-one others.

A group of policemen guarding Murari Gas Station opened up to me.

'There are more than 500 people here. We understand their anguish. With hospitals turning them away and the government refusing to allow them to get oxygen from the plants, their miseries have doubled,' one of them lamented. 'Our hands are tied. We have been given orders to prevent them from entering the gas stations.'

Twenty-two-year-old Amritanshu Pandey, who had travelled from Jankipuram in Lucknow to the gas station, approached the policeman I was talking to. His father, Sukhdev Pandey's oxygen saturation had fallen below 60. Amritanshu hadn't been able to secure a hospital bed for him; he was isolating at home.

'We rushed from one gas station to another, but none would refill the cylinder,' Amritanshu told me. 'In Lucknow, every hospital bed equipped with oxygen supply is occupied. There is no help.'

Even the elderly stood in queues for oxygen, hospital beds or tests for hours. Elderly couples, with their children living in faraway cities and countries, were particularly vulnerable. It was the worst time to be alone.

M.D. Singh, stood in the same queue as Amritanshu Pandey. He lived on the bustling Cantt Road with his wife Aruna Singh, aged seventy-six. She was COVID-positive and had a history of diabetes. He stood crying, watching young and old men lifting heavy steel and aluminium cylinders into cars and onto bikes to run to another gas station.

Experts criticised the government's directive to deny oxygen to those who were isolated in homes as 'arbitrary'. There was no merit in the order, many said. Dr A.K. Shukla, a former Chief Medical Officer, described it as a 'blanket order'.

'Halting oxygen supply to individuals is a bad decision,' he asserted. 'It's not just COVID patients who need oxygen but also those with asthma. Where will they go? The government should reconsider its order.'

Despite the government taking the most stringent measures to direct oxygen through official channels, the crisis had reached a point where even hospitals did not receive the necessary high flow oxygen. Across the city, ambulances waited at the gates of oxygen plants and supply agencies. Hospital administrators raised alarms when their stock ran out.

Nishant Singh, the manager at Make Well Hospital in Gomti Nagar, said 'We have appealed to the government that if they can provide half the number of oxygen cylinders we need, we will try to procure the rest. But there has been no assistance. Even our regular vendors are out of oxygen. We have had to put shortage notices on our gates.'

Charak Hospital faced a similar dilemma. 'The oxygen crisis hasn't been resolved yet. It has paralysed our efforts,' Suparna Dutta, a staff member went on record.

Ultimately, hospitals had to shut their doors to new patients even when beds were vacant.

At the beginning of May, an Allahabad High Court bench comprising Justice Siddharth Verma and Justice Ajit Kumar took cognizance of the shortage of oxygen. 'We are pained at observing that COVID patients have died due to short supply of oxygen in hospitals. It is a criminal act and no less than a genocide by those who have been entrusted with the task of ensuring continuous procurement and supply chain of liquid medical oxygen.'[2] The state reacted only when made aware of the outrage on social media.

For instance, in UP, the orders and notices were released on Twitter before being sent in the form of official communication from the state to the concerned departments. When CM Yogi Adityanath tweeted that symptomatic patients would also be admitted, I went to some hospitals to check if they were indeed admitting symptomatic patients. Most hospitals said that it was a tweet, not an order. They waited for it to turn into an official, written order.

Over the years, we have seen how the state has skillfully used social media and the pandemic was no different. When it came to concrete results, outcomes fell severely short of expectations. The then UP Health Minister, Jai Pratap Singh, assured that the state was taking the necessary measures to overcome the oxygen crisis. 'All hospitals will have adequate oxygen supply very soon,' he said. Chief Minister Yogi Adityanath, taking a firm stand against the illicit trading of oxygen, warned that those caught selling oxygen on the black market would be prosecuted under the National Security Act (NSA).[3]

According to a report by the *BBC*, India's healthcare facilities typically accounted for 15 per cent of the country's oxygen consumption, leaving majority of the share—85 per cent—for industrial use. But during the second wave, nearly 90 per cent of the country's oxygen was redirected for medical care. In response to the crisis, the Indian government allocated 7,500 metric tonnes of oxygen per day to healthcare consumption.[4]

After the first wave, the central health ministry had allocated a budget of 201.58 crores to set up new oxygen plants.[5] In October 2020, it invited bids for 162 pressure swing adsorption (PSA) plants across the country.[6]

However, by the time the second wave hit, only thirty-three had been installed. The government tweeted that fifty-nine more would be installed by the end of April, and the remaining eighty by the end of May.[7]

As during the migrant exodus, 'Shramik' trains were flagged off to send people back to their home states, trains named 'Oxygen Express' were started in order to deliver Liquid Medical Oxygen (LMO) tankers to hospitals across India. First, Madhya Pradesh and Maharashtra sought critical assistance from Indian Railways, and then Uttar Pradesh joined in.

The Indian Railways dispatched its second 'Oxygen Express' from Lucknow carrying seven–eight empty tankers to Jharkhand's Bokaro to collect liquid medical oxygen.

The Ministry of Railways said that between 19 April and mid-May, 130 Oxygen Express trains delivered over 8,700 tonnes of liquid medical oxygen in more than 540 tankers to oxygen-starved states. When this data was released, there were six Oxygen Express trains on their way to various states with 475 metric tonnes of liquid medical oxygen in thirty-five tankers.[8]

The Indian Air Force was also mobilised to airlift oxygen supplies from military installations, importing 50,000 metric tonnes of liquid oxygen.[9]

The Union Health Ministry issued a statement that said the government was also floating a tender for importing 50,000 million metric tonnes of medical oxygen; the Ministry of External Affairs was tasked with exploring possible sources.[10]

So desperate measures were taken to counter the acute oxygen crisis. However, when it came to documenting COVID deaths due to lack of oxygen, there is no official data available. It was later revealed that in the medical reports issued during the second wave, oxygen shortage wasn't cited as a cause of death. The deaths were, instead, attributed to co-morbidities.

In the Parliament sessions that followed the second wave, the government informed the House that no COVID deaths had been reported due to the lack of oxygen supply. This happened first in July 2021, when Bharati Pravin Pawar, minister of state, health and family welfare, told the Rajya Sabha that no deaths due to lack of oxygen had been specifically reported by the states and union territories.[11] His response came in reply to Congress MP K.C. Venugopal, who asked whether it was true that many patients had died on roads and in hospitals due to shortage of oxygen; he also asked what steps the government had taken afterwards to ensure that there would be no scarcity during the imminent third wave of infections.

The government reiterated this stance when a similar question was asked in the Parliament six months later. In Uttar Pradesh, the state government aligned with the central government—in the legislative council, Health Minister Jai Pratap Singh claimed that the state had issued 22,915 death certificates and none of them mentioned lack of oxygen as the cause of death.[12]

The migrant exodus during the first wave and the oxygen crisis during the second wave were largely unmitigated disasters that warrant continued scrutiny.

In 2025, when the Civil Registration System (CRS) report was finally released, the journalists who had covered the second wave stood vindicated.[13]

For people, who had long suspected the undercounting, the ORGI report was a confirmation of the truth. Excess deaths (the difference between the total number of deaths in 2020–21 and the average death rate of the previous years) in 2021 alone, were nearly six times higher than the officially reported COVID-19 deaths.

Some states were disproportionately affected by the underreporting of COVID deaths. For instance, in the case of states like Gujarat, Madhya Pradesh and Uttar Pradesh, the number of excess deaths far exceeded the respective official COVID-19 fatality figures.

The undercounting left a vast population deprived of the state's attention. They received neither relief nor compensation.

7

The Doms

The next leg of my journey took me to Varanasi. The ancient city, surrounded by Jaunpur, Mirzapur, Ghazipur, Chandauli and Bhadohi, happens to be the constituency of Prime Minister Narendra Modi.

Having driven about 300 kilometres from Lucknow, we were now in the city lanes, looking for a hotel. Smaller hotels had shut shop after facing massive financial losses. Only a few remained unexpectedly functional with reduced staff. It didn't take us long to find a decent one on Cantonment Road. Varanasi, just like Lucknow, Prayagraj and Gorakhpur, was grappling with the worst infrastructure breakdown. The deaths were too many to count. The city's crematoriums worked day and night and its hospitals, including the prestigious Banaras Hindu University Medical College Hospital, were overstretched.

District reporters, local leaders and activists had retreated into their homes. Ground reporters weren't able to travel to gather stories. As a result, the rural belts remained veiled in silence.

What was the story of the rest of India beyond the pyres burning in the cities? This question led me towards a new chapter in my assignment.

IT cell trolls had launched a scathing campaign against those of us who reported from the ground, holding us responsible for 'spreading negativity'. They branded us as 'vultures' (drawing parallels between the iconic 1993 Kevin Carter photograph of a collapsed child lying vulnerably close to a vulture during the famine in Sudan).

With every report that went live, the IT cell flooded the comment sections of the handles of journalists like Danish Siddiqui, me and many others reporting from the frontlines.

The Uttar Pradesh government had also grown increasingly antagonistic following the reports on undercounting of deaths. In Varanasi, the stakes were even higher. As the constituency of Prime Minister Narendra Modi, any news coming from the ground was subjected to intense scrutiny.

The evening I reached Varanasi was marked by the haunting images of the Ganga ghats. The visuals had gone viral, sending shockwaves across social media platforms. I visited the Manikarnika and Raja Harishchandra ghats that very evening. Countless dead bodies were there. Long queues of corpses awaited their last rites. Those who had spent their entire lives at these ghats—the shopkeepers, labourers, Doms (cremators) and priests—all said they had never witnessed anything of this magnitude.

The state wanted to divert the media's gaze from the ghats. The Varanasi district administration, in a strategic move, established a makeshift tin crematorium overnight, and called it Ramana Ghat. This new ghat was located on the opposite bank of the Ganga river. The counterparts of Varanasi's local administration in Lucknow had blocked the burning pyres from sight by installing tin sheds. Since I had already reported on the undercounting of deaths from Lucknow, I decided not to pursue the same line in another city.

Instead, I returned to my hotel and sent emails and messages to the Collector, CMO and other key officials, seeking appointments to have a word with them. The next morning, I started visiting their offices in person, but in vain.

Disappointed, I returned to Harishchandra Ghat that evening. As I entered the narrow alleys, a group of Doms was carrying a body to its final destination. I trailed after it. The Doms had severely tanned bodies, and their eyes were red. Their gamchhas were soaked in sweat. They paid no heed to my camera.

Unlike the doctors, the nurses and the bureaucrats, who had taken centre stage as frontline soldiers, the Doms remained in the shadows. They wore no gloves, masks or PPE kits. No relief packages were announced for them.

They toiled silently in the crematoriums along the Ganga. They carried the dead who had been abandoned on their last journey by their families. Their contribution during the second wave went unnoticed by a large section of the media and the administration. What does this oversight tell us?

That the first draft of history systemically excluded a particular community?

As the group of Doms vanished into the smoke rising from the burning pyres, I spotted the person in charge of Harishchandra Ghat at a distance. He was busy making phone calls as his role involved coordination between the Nagar Nigam and the Doms at the cremation ground. We sat down nearby to talk about the situation.

He started with an incident when his team of young men had cremated the corpse of an elderly lady whose family hadn't turned up for the last rites. Then he pointed towards a group of Doms: 'Some of them went to her home and carried her here.'

This wasn't their duty to perform as they weren't formally employed by the Nagar Nigam. But since the Nagar Nigam across the country was struggling with human resources, they outsourced some of the work to these Doms.

I later verified the incident with an official in the local administration. He had been tasked with the duty of getting the abandoned corpses cremated.

'There are families that simply refuse to come forward for the last rites. At BHU, this is an everyday occurrence. We wait for some time and then call the Doms,' he said. But the Doms weren't paid a penny for the extra mile they went to provide people dignity in death. They were overworked, underpaid and exhausted.

My source revealed that the elderly lady was related to a civil servant who was then serving as secretary in a central ministry.

'Actually,' he paused, 'the district magistrate (Kaushal Raj Sharma) received a call from New Delhi. The mother or mother-in-law of a senior IAS officer was living in the city all by herself. A cook used to look after her. The officer from New Delhi requested a team of doctors to check on her since they hadn't heard from her for quite some time. The Collector assigned this task to the Chief Medical Officer (CMO).' When the team arrived at her house, they discovered that she had passed away.

'The Collector contacted the secretary and both, the CMO and the Collector, patiently waited for the family to come and take charge of the last rites. But when the secretary said the last rites should proceed without his family's presence, the Doms were called in,' he added.

When I discovered the identity of the secretary, I sent him a condolence message, 'I am sorry for your loss. I heard about your close relative in Varanasi.' The secretary never responded. I also refrained from pursuing the story.

Hundreds of families hesitated to go to crematoriums during the second wave, fearing the viral load in hospitals or worrying for their family members who were still uninfected. However, the kind of apathy some families displayed towards their elderly members is indescribable. In a viral video recorded by a Noida-based hospital's staff member, one family denied entry to their recovered grandmother. The hospital team stood outside their home, waiting for access. Eventually, one of them had to scale the gate to open it from the inside.

I closely followed the Doms while in Varanasi. They worked in gruelling twelve to fifteen-hour shifts every day without breaking to eat. The break only came at night when they sat down after cremating the last corpse in the queue. Getting a conversation with them during the day proved nearly impossible. Even if some of them did speak to me, the exchanges lacked depth. So, I kept following them through narrow alleys right up to the entrance of the burning ghats, interjecting with questions along the way. At night, they would gather on the steps by the riverbank, and consume locally-made liquor to cope with physical and emotional exhaustion.

When I briefed him about my story, Arunesh had unequivocally declared that he would not drive me to the ghats after dark.

His reluctance came from a genuine concern for me. 'If you were a man, I wouldn't hesitate to drive you around at midnight. But it's not safe for you.' One of my daytime trips to the Ganga acquainted me with Akash Chaudhary (name changed to protect identity), a thin and sharp-faced Dom in his late twenties. I requested him to sit with me for a bit. Though initially hesitant, he joined me near a pyre assigned to him, as it demanded his undivided attention. He had to finish the cremation as quickly as he could because the next corpse, shrouded in white and with a marigold garland over it, awaited him.

'What can we do? We are not even getting time to have a proper meal. If it weren't for the liquor, how would we light so many pyres?' He continued, 'Since the priests have fled, the Doms have to perform their duty as well.'

'How many bodies have you cremated in a single day?' I asked.

'Thirty-five,' he counted on his fingertips.

'Since when have you been at this ghat?'

'Since childhood. I don't even remember when I began cremating bodies.'

I prodded further, 'Have you ever seen these many bodies before?'

'Never. It takes hours to cremate one body. Burning pyres non-stop over the years in scorching sun has burnt my body.' He wiped off sweat from his forehead. The corpse's head still needed more heat. Akash waited for the head to turn into ashes as his team climbed the stairs to bring in another COVID body abandoned by its family.

The surroundings of the ghat buzzed with people, some wearing double masks, others with face shields and a few in full PPE suits. The usual legacy Banarasi sari shops stood shuttered. Only vendors selling shrouds, garlands and wood for pyres and a handful of tea stalls remained open.

Close to where Akash and I sat, a tea vendor was resting. A mother and her daughter were mourning their dead silently, standing on one side; the daughter adjusted her mask and gloves while the mother stared into the void. Families had no time to come to terms with the sudden demise of their loved ones. And then they jostled at the ghats to find space for cremation.

During the first wave, the Indian government had permitted the participation of twenty relatives in the funeral of a non-COVID deceased; only five people could attend the cremation in case of a COVID-related death. The second wave changed the rules. Now, some bodies arrived with a few attendants, while some came with none. In Delhi, where the crematoriums ran out of space, people had to cremate their relatives in parking lots and along the sides of roads. The pandemic challenged the practices that had gone on for generations. For instance, women aren't traditionally allowed to light funeral pyres. But at Harishchandra Ghat, I witnessed a mother-daughter duo standing side by side in front of a pyre. With trembling hands, they lit the pyre of their loved one. The Doms, who had carried the corpse on the deceased's final journey, stepped forward to assume the role of a priest, guiding the pair. For me, as a woman, witnessing this scene where both women and Doms defied centuries-old norms was surreal.

Meanwhile, at Manikarnika Ghat, located 2.5 km away from Harishchandra Ghat, a young man called his elder brother, who lived in a distant city, on WhatsApp and they conducted the last rites for their father virtually. The traditions had shifted not just for COVID deaths but also for non-COVID ones.

The usual thirteen-day shradh ceremonies couldn't be performed within homes, people couldn't be invited in.

I spoke to an elderly shopkeeper who sold wood for funeral pyres about the rituals observed in regular times.

'Usually, the corpse is bathed to cleanse both the body and the soul. But now the COVID-infected body arrives shrouded in a polythene bag. The family isn't supposed to touch the body,' he explained.

'Both the Doms and the priests fled the ghats during the initial chaos. But the Doms returned. Normally, it's priests who chant sacred verses during the lighting of the pyre. Now, the task to perform the rituals had fallen upon the Doms.'

The images emerging from these ghats shook the government which had previously declared victory over the pandemic and conducted election rallies and the Kumbh Mela.

After staring into the waters of the Ganga for a while, I climbed the stairs leading up to the electric crematorium designated for COVID victims. The machines stood idle, their walls and tin roofs charred and swallowed by blackness.

'Machino ko bhi aaram chahiye.' (Even the machines need rest), Dilip Chaudhary (name changed to protect identity), a senior Dom, commented.

'What is there to feel about death? We were born here. We see death every day,' Dilip's voice carried the weight of generations.

'For the past fifteen days, we've worked in the haze of intoxication.' Beside him lay the death register, a record of the lives lost.

People were now mere ink on paper. As I stood with my camera in the middle of the electric crematorium, Dilip counted aloud,

'Twenty-one, twenty-two, twenty-three … madam, on 17 April, we received twenty-three bodies.'

The acrid smell of death and the extreme heat emanating from the furnaces made it hard for me to stand beneath that roof. So, I stepped out in the open copying data from his register into my notebook.

Arunesh awaited my return at the end of the narrow alleys. He had been quite patient with my investigations, but not on that day. He had almost brawled with a drunk.

I couldn't resist saying, 'Kya Arunesh-ji, ab aap sharabi aadmi se bhi nahi nipat sakte?' (Arunesh ji, can't you handle one drunk?)

'Arey madam …' His response was a mix of exasperation and amusement. I pulled up Google Maps to find the location of the makeshift Ramana Ghat. As we drove off, I checked my inbox. My emails and messages to the CMO, Collector, ADM and SDMs remained unanswered.

*The caste name, Dom, has been used in relation to the profession of the community. The intention is not to identify specific people or use their caste identity as a pejorative.

8

Dying Like Flies: A Tale of Two Varanasi Villages

My editor Rama Lakshmi always tells me that in order to craft a powerful narrative, you should become a fly on the wall.

So, around 11 p.m., I dialled Arunesh, requesting him to accompany me to the ghats again. He bluntly refused, 'Ever since we started from Lucknow, you have only been visiting cremation grounds.'

Those familiar with lead, nut graph or a big-picture quote for ground reports would understand the challenge I faced. I wanted to capture the Doms sitting on the ghats or near the pyres at midnight, pondering the tragedy or maybe having a quiet drink. This is what they told me they did after cremating the last corpse of the day.

I wanted to begin my report with their solitary moments. Since Arunesh wasn't keen on visiting the ghats at night, I decided to visit the Doms for the last time during the day.

But the next morning, I received a call from the Lucknow cab service. Arunesh no longer wished to continue with me on the assignment.

'He is complaining that you have been visiting too many crematoriums. He wants to return to his family.'

Since Arunesh felt uncomfortable going to the crematoriums, so I decided to explore nearby villages instead.

This was the last week of April. The country was recording nearly 400,000 new cases and mourning over 3,000 deaths each day.[1] The world's critical gaze was fixed on us.

International media giants such as *Al Jazeera*, Channel 4, and DW sent their reporters to Varanasi.

Since I was already reporting from there, the primetime anchors of international channels sought my insights for their shows. As I sat across from them in a corner of my hotel room, fixing the light and mic, they probed me. Unfortunately, they cared more about their headlines than the heartbreaks my stories carried.

In Varanasi, a story appeared on the third page of a local daily without a byline. Two villages had seen two dozen deaths within a fortnight. The story carried names of villagers accompanied by official statements from the district administration. The cause of deaths was apparently a mystery.

I was intrigued. We left the city to go to Tilamapur and Ashapur in Chiraigaon block of Varanasi district.

It was a Sunday afternoon. Since the UP government had imposed a weekend lockdown in the state, the roads that otherwise teemed with bicycles and rickshaws lay deserted, and shops were shuttered. Both villages were twenty-five km away from the main city. As we neared the villages, I saw a grand house in Chiraigaon with big cars parked outside and people moving through the iron gate. I thought it belonged to a local politician, maybe an MLA. I asked Arunesh to stop the car so I could take a closer look.

I approached the entrance, the nameplate said 'Sudhir Singh'. I later found out that Sudhir Singh's wife was the Block Pramukh. He was a Bahubali, but he was no longer operating the way he once did. The state government's crackdown on Bahubalis across UP had forced him to change tactics, retreating from the spotlight. His wife, the officially elected Block Pramukh, now held the title, but it was his authority that continued to dictate regional affairs.

I hurried towards the office where a few men sat across a table from a tall man with gold rings on every finger and thumb.

Sudhir Singh was on the phone. His subordinates checked my ID and whispered something to him. I found a spot and sat down. The men watched me with curiosity as we all waited for Sudhir to finish his phone call. 'Take Zinc,' he advised the person on the other side of the call. 'Paracetamol will be available somewhere. Check your WhatsApp—I'm sending you the medicine list.' Another phone rang as soon as he hung up. He seemed to have multiple phones.

Each call seemed to be a plea for help.

'Boliye … arre koi hospital nahin le raha hai Varanasi mein. Kya lakshan hain? Bukhar aa raha hai? Yeh dawa lena shuru kijiye. Koi madad nahin kar raha hai abhi, samajhiye,' he instructed another caller. (No hospital is admitting patients in Varanasi. What symptoms are you experiencing? Fever? Get these medicines. Please understand, there's no one to assist.)

He then gestured to his subordinate and within minutes, tea was arranged for. Meanwhile, Sudhir kept answering calls.

My initial impression was that he was a doctor saving lives through tele-consultation, but he clarified that he wasn't one. The calls came from the villages nearby. When no help came from medical institutions, he would get a physician to write a prescription for someone in need. Or if a villager called him for help, he would ask about symptoms and then prescribe basic medicines. This was the only way he thought he could save lives.

'People are dying like flies in the villages,' he said. 'I haven't had time to eat, I receive over a hundred phone calls every day for hospital beds and consultations. There is no hope. No doctors are available and we are losing our young generation to this disease.'

He continued to shed light on the rural crisis: 'Things got worse after 19 April when the block went to the panchayat polls. The number of calls seeking help has increased drastically. During the polls, the candidates contesting for elections called back their loyal voters from Gujarat, Delhi, Maharashtra, etc. But they weren't tested or screened when they arrived. Now, in every village, patients are grappling with fever and pneumonia.'

Two men entered the room just then and complained of fever. They had travelled a fair distance. Sudhir's subordinates ran to bring masks and directed the two men to go to the adjacent room.

A few minutes later, I got up to leave for Tilamapur and Ashapur. Luckily, Sudhir Singh gave me the contact numbers of both the village heads.

On our way to Tilamapur, I contacted the village head, forty-six–year–old Satish Mishra, and the first thing he said was that it was his wife who officially held the position of village head, but being the husband, he unofficially handled all the responsibilities, not uncommon in villages across India. The Indian state may have reserved seats for women at the panchayat level, but their participation remains low. It is often their husbands, fathers-in-law or brothers-in-law who tackle the actual work. In many parts of north India, they are known as 'Pradhan Pati', 'Pradhan Jeth' or 'Pradhan Sasur'.

Mishra said he hadn't maintained a record of the deaths in his village.

'But I receive news of a death in the village every day. Without COVID testing, the cause of these mysterious deaths remains unknown.'

I pressed for more information.

'All these deaths were among individuals who experienced fever, cough and breathing difficulties,' Mishra said in a low voice. He sounded unwell.

I asked if I could visit him. His initial response was that he himself had a high fever, cough and body ache. When I insisted that it was crucial for my assignment that I meet him, he gave me permission.

We arrived at his two-storey ancestral home. Two workers were painting its time-worn iron gate. I dialled Mishra's number to let him know that I had arrived. The call went unanswered. As I waited outside the gate, one of the workers popped outside to tell me, 'Ek hafte se oopar waale kamre mein rehte hain. Kisi se nahi milte hain.' (He has been staying in the upstairs room for over a week now. He doesn't meet anyone.)

I decided to wait outside the gate. I stood melting in the scorching summer heat, wearing three masks. Just when my patience was about to run out, Mishra called back.

'I have confined myself to the second story of my house for the past week. I've been self-isolating and taking the COVID kit medicines,' he said.

He told me that like many of his fellow villagers, he hadn't yet taken a COVID test. I asked him why he, the one who called all the shots in the village, hadn't taken the test yet, but he didn't have a specific reason.

In Tilamapur, one of the 1,258 villages in the Varanasi district, only a few residents ventured out due to the heat or fear of infection. The usual card-playing group of elderly men, the giggles of children playing in the backyards and the sounds of women chatting, were all missing.

When I started knocking on doors, I found that at least one family member in each household had a fever and cough.

The adjoining Ashapur village had witnessed over a dozen deaths in the last fifteen days, all attributed to 'fever and cough'.

When I managed to trace the house of the village head in Ashapur—Santosh Pandey—it was filled with people who ran a fever. To avoid contact, we sat outside the main house, in an airy verandah.

'Even the young are succumbing to this illness. Recently, forty-year-old Kailash Tripathi and his wife lost their lives to a fever. Rafiqer's wife and son also passed away from similar symptoms.

People soon began to realise that these deaths were connected to the Coronavirus. During the last wave, we dismissed it as some kind of conspiracy. But now it's painfully real. Even thirty-year-olds are not spared. Thirteen people must've died by now,' said Santosh Pandey.

Varanasi was one of the four worst-affected districts in Uttar Pradesh, and Uttar Pradesh was the second worst-affected state in the country, with more than 2.97 lakh active COVID cases. But the official death toll did not account for the realities of villages such as Tilamapur and Ashapur. On 25 April, Varanasi's district health bulletin reported only eight COVID-related deaths.

The block where the villages were located had one community health centre (CHC) and four primary health centres (PHCs). To gain deeper insights into rural healthcare, I visited the CHC in Narayanpur village. The building appeared to be abandoned. There wasn't a single person in sight, but a few ambulances were parked within the premises. Some residents nearby informed me that the CHC had been shut since the second wave hit in late March.

So, where were the residents getting tested and accessing medication? Not everyone could afford private facilities, many of which were also shut. Through a source in the COVID management team in the district, I accessed the figures from an internal report sent to the Lucknow Headquarters.

According to this report, out of the four PHCs, only one was actively collecting samples for COVID testing in the entire block. The numbers were worrying. Only 107 samples were tested on 17 April, followed by zero from 18 to 20 April. 197 samples were tested on 21–22 April, and 147 samples on 23 April.

A few kilometres away from the CHC stood the PHC that collected these samples. A poster announcing that COVID-19 samples were collected for testing between 10 a.m. and noon hung on its main gate. Outside the PHC, there was a police vehicle. A few policemen and a staffer, Dinesh Kumar, stood inside the testing room. Dinesh informed me, 'On Sundays, the centre remains closed.' 'We test 100–150 people every day,' he added.

In Chiraigaon block, not far from the historical site of Sarnath—one among the holiest Buddhist pilgrimages—a vibrant tourist culture once thrived. There used to be educational institutes, temples, overbridges, marriage gardens, bars and hotels everywhere in this area.

But being a tourist destination did not guarantee a robust healthcare infrastructure. The block, which comprises 137 villages and a population of 2.31 lakh, faced significant challenges when it came to testing. Even lady village heads and their husbands had to resort to self-isolation because there were no other solutions available.

After visiting the CHC and PHCs, I started touring the emergency private hospitals in the block. One of them, Meridian Hospital, was entirely shut. On its gate was a notice announcing 'No beds and oxygen available'. I called the owner, who said the hospital had not received authorisation from the Varanasi Collector to function as a COVID facility.

A few kilometres away from Meridian Hospital was another private facility called Smart Medicity Hospital. It was functioning with just two ventilators and ten oxygen beds.

Dr Deepak Singh, who was monitoring the two patients on ventilators, said, 'Last week, we faced an acute shortage of oxygen supply. We cannot admit more patients and risk their lives.'

V.P. Singh, the CMO of Varanasi, lost his ninety-year-old father to COVID. So, when Singh was on leave, Dr S.S. Kannaujiya, the additional chief medical officer, and district surveillance officer for COVID-19, stepped in.

I called Dr Kannaujiya to get clarity on the low testing figures. 'We are actively conducting COVID tests at the Primary Health Center (PHC), and our COVID sampling teams are also reaching out to villages. But due to the block's proximity to the main city, many people are opting to get tested at Banaras Hindu University (BHU) and other authorised testing centres.'

I asked him about the deaths in Tilamapur and Ashapur villages. He acknowledged the number of deaths but not the cause.

'Unless the deceased's report is positive for COVID, we cannot officially count it as a COVID related death,' he said firmly.

My story was published on 27 April 2021 with the headline, 'The young in these 2 Varanasi villages started to die. That's when Covid became "real"'.[2] I am not certain about the impact of the report, but about a month after I returned to New Delhi, I received an email from someone who credited my report with saving their grandparents' lives. The email said that after the story went viral on social media, his family managed timely intervention for the elderly couple who lived alone in a village in Varanasi.

The virus had ignited not just fear but also stigma in the villages. In Tilamapur village, I met the family of twenty-three-year-old Akash Mishra. Akash used to work as a sales officer with HDFC Bank in Varanasi, but returned home when the lockdown was announced in 2020 and never went back to the city.

He spoke to me through his closed front gate.

On 8 April, his father had complained of chest pain. Akash's family promptly sent his samples for testing, but the results did not arrive in time. By 12 April, his oxygen levels had dropped to 60, and he passed away on his way to the hospital. His report arrived later that night; he was COVID positive.

Akash showed me his father's last photos on his phone. The villagers who learned of his father's diagnosis refrained from offering condolences. It was quite unusual for a rural household to be left alone to mourn. The stigma surrounding COVID-19 became deeply entrenched in the rural society. Even after the recommended quarantine period, Akash's neighbours continued to keep their distance.

Akash was bewildered at why block officials had failed to advise the family to isolate or get themselves tested.

'We took it upon ourselves to isolate for fourteen days after his death and took all the prescribed medicines for Covid.'

Just a few metres away from Akash Mishra's house lived Santosh Mishra's family. Santosh, just forty-eight, had died on 9 April. His family and relatives were reluctant to disclose the details of his death. But when I disclosed my identity, one of his uncles opened up.

Santosh was diabetic and he complained of breathlessness on 9 April.

'When all our efforts to secure an oxygen cylinder failed, we rushed him to Ashirvad Hospital. It is only two km away from the village. But he could not make it.' The hospital refused to admit him, resulting in no COVID test or post-mortem examination.

'Santosh, then, isn't a COVID victim because we have no piece of paper that says he was infected,' said his uncle. Their twenty-three–member joint family decided to get tested at the block testing centre a few days after Santosh's death. Their antigen tests all came out negative.

Other families were too fearful to admit that their loved one's death had something to do with COVID symptoms. Coming at it from a social angle, I think the virus affected different sections of people differently. The tale of two families of Tilamapur village and the unseen lives of Doms were just two examples.

While Akash managed to send his father's COVID-19 samples, Santosh's family failed to arrange an oxygen cylinder. Factors such as class, caste, region, age and even gender shaped individual experiences. As someone rightly said, it all depended on who you were and where you were.

9

The Returned Migrants in Jaunpur

The distress that I observed in the two Varanasi villages led me to expand my investigation into the neighbouring district of Jaunpur. Situated around sixty-five km from Varanasi, this district in Purvanchal has 92 per cent of its population living in rural areas.

Despite its closeness to the rapidly developing city of Varanasi, it struggles with education, healthcare and basic infrastructure.

Arunesh had decided to stay back with me after I stopped visiting the ghats. I found out that, Sajid Ali, my colleague from the video team, had also arrived in Varanasi by then to document the crisis. He had been producing videos from the burning ghats when he decided to accompany me to Jaunpur.

Our first stop was the district hospital—named after Amar Shaheed Umanath Singh, a prominent Jaunpur leader who had served as Jail Minister in 1991, by the Yogi Adityanath government.

The hospital was near Jaunpur Railway Junction. Patients with symptoms were coming in droves, oxygen cylinders were being rushed here and there, clueless attendants scurried in all directions seeking medicines for their sick relatives. Amidst this chaos, I made my way to the chock-a-block emergency ward where patients lay on stretchers and even on the floor, gasping for air.

Seventy-year-old Bamau Ram Kannojia's oxygen mask had slipped off his nose. His eyes searched the room for a familiar face.

His wrinkled hands trembled. A young man of twenty-five, holding documents wrapped in a plastic bag, approached the stretcher. He told me he was a distant relative. We called out to the nursing staff. A male staffer came and readjusted the mask before disappearing into the crowd to attend to other patients.

'How did he get infected?' I asked the young man. Ticking off a mental checklist to identify the source of Kannojia's infection, the relative said, 'He never stepped outside the village, mostly stayed indoors. How can he get COVID? We have no idea.'

Kannojia was among the fourteen critical patients on oxygen support in the ward. None had ever left their villages.

When a doctor arrived, Kannojia rattled off all his symptoms but added that his biggest worry was neither the fever nor the breathlessness but how he would eat. 'Baaki sab toh theek hai, bukhar nahi ja raha, saans nahi aa rahi, khana kaise khaaunga?' The rest is fine but the fever hasn't subsided and I can't breathe. How will I eat?'

'Soon,' the doctor reassured him, 'you will eat once you recover.'

A Muslim family rushed in, their daughter-in-law struggling to breathe. She was immediately put on oxygen support. Her anxious husband ran to the OPD adjacent to the emergency ward where a long queue of people was waiting to be examined.

Inside the room, two doctors carefully recorded each patient's symptoms. Many attendants here were without a mask.

Six-seven patients died every day here, with their deaths not officially attributed to COVID-19 as they could not be tested or even attended to in time, the doctors told me.

In the span of just sixteen days, Jaunpur—a district with twenty-one administrative blocks and 747 villages—found itself dealing with a massive surge in cases—from 867 active COVID cases on 11 April to 5,000 by 27 April. There was a surge of 476.6 per cent.

COVID, on the ascent again after a dip in infections, was moving into the rural belt now in all its fury. Jaunpur had one Level 1 government hospital equipped with isolation beds (so they could tend to patients with mild symptoms) and four Level 2 hospitals with oxygen beds. But none of these hospitals had ventilators. At that critical juncture, the district only had twenty-eight ventilator equipped hospital beds.

The district administration had recruited six private hospitals to bolster its healthcare infrastructure, and even then there were just 598 isolation, oxygen and ventilator beds put together for a population of 4.49 million.

The administration tried to understand the reason for the rural surge. One explanation that District Magistrate Manish Kumar Verma offered was the influx of returning migrants. In Jaunpur alone, as many as 1 lakh migrants had returned from various parts of the country before Holi (29 March 2021).

'People started coming for Holi, then for the harvest, and then for panchayat polls. Overall, one lakh migrants have returned to the district,' said Verma.

Though no Collector or other officials across the state directly blamed the Panchayat polls, many of them told me off-the-record that the polls were a disaster, for not only keeping officials, who would have otherwise taken care of pandemic management, engaged in poll duty but also for becoming a superspreader event as thousands gathered not on just the counting day but also on the polling day.

The polls were originally supposed to be held in November–December 2020 but were postponed due to the pandemic and eventually held in four phases from 15 April to 19 April 2021, right in the thick of the deadly second wave.[1]

Jaunpur voted in the first phase. I spoke to Anil Yadav, a former head of Chaktali village in Gaddi Pur gram panchayat, about six km away from the district headquarters. Chaktali was a small village with a hundred households.

'We never received any directives to prepare for the returned migrants. They continued to arrive, but there was neither screening nor testing. From the gram sabhas to the district administration, no one was prepared,' said Yadav, who was the village head until December 2020. Manoj Yadav, former village head of Gohka gram panchayat, corroborated this. His panchayat was forty kilometres away from Jaunpur city. He claimed that despite not being the official head anymore, he oversaw the crisis management in his personal capacity.

Unlike their active involvement during the initial outbreak, the village heads were exempted from COVID-19 management responsibilities after December 2020. During the first wave, they had worked closely with multiple stakeholders to address the migrant exodus, establish quarantine facilities at the panchayat level and manage the distribution of food, masks, sanitisers and other essentials.

'After our tenure ends, we do not hold administrative responsibilities. Now, it is primarily the ASHA (Accredited Social Health Activists) workers and Anganwadi staff, along with the block development officers (BDOs), who are taking the lead in the second wave,' said Manoj Yadav. The Panchayat poll results were to be announced on 2 May. The district authorities kept pinning the blame on the migrants for not self-isolating and thus causing the surge. While the state, despite the severity of the crisis, went right ahead and conducted the elections.

Anita Yadav, an Anganwadi worker from Chaktali village, said that Anganwadi workers initially did not receive any instructions to monitor the returning migrants.

'It wasn't until after 10 April that the administration issued directives. As a result, those who had already returned before this date were not subjected to checks or screening simply because we were not asked to monitor them,' she explained. The Anganwadi workers swung into action only after 11 April.

'From that day on, we've been keeping a register, conducting door-to-door visits, and urging villagers to get tested at the block health centre,' Anita added.

However, the migrants were reluctant to disclose their symptoms, making it hard for Anganwadi workers like Anita. The fear and stigma posed a great challenge to the testing efforts.

I tracked down a returned migrant in Chatkali. Bhaiyalal Yadav, a daily wage worker who made his way back from Mumbai on 14 April.

'They took my temperature at the Allahabad railway station. After clearing the screening, I boarded a bus to my village. When I reached the village, some Anganwadi workers came to conduct a health check. I assured them that I had no symptoms,' he said.

Then I checked with another migrant, who had returned before 10 April and no one had approached him for screening or testing. Both the migrants ratified Anita Yadav's account.

To track the movement of over a lakh returned migrants was daunting for the district administration. By the time, they were traced, they could have transmitted the virus to numerous individuals in their villages.

To curb the spread of the virus, the district administration divided Jaunpur into more than 500 containment zones, covering both urban and rural areas. District Magistrate Verma elaborated on their strategy of 'smart testing'.

'We are doing targeted testing. We are prioritising those who are at a higher risk of exposure to the virus, such as street vendors and migrants returning from COVID hotspots,' he explained. The administration also set up 1,740 nigrani samitis (surveillance committees) in the villages and 164 in urban pockets. Each committee comprised an ASHA and an Anganwadi worker, among others, to monitor susceptible individuals and alert the authorities. These committees were not only tasked with vigilant tracking but were also given medical kits to distribute. The kits had recommended medication.

My story on Jaunpur's rural surge was published a day later, but the fact that we managed to acquire official statistics and internal reports from the COVID Command Centre was no small feat.

Since the district administration's top officials were cautious of sharing information with journalists, the COVID Command Centre came to our rescue. Sajid and I, just drove there and sneaked in. Sajid's appearance and foreign accent made a favourable impression on the officials in the room and they spoke freely.

There were multiple unwarranted FIRs registered against journalists for either sharing viral videos or leaking crucial statistics, and we didn't want any trouble.

My fears were not unfounded. Nearly a week after our visit, the Jaunpur administration filed an FIR against a local reporter. His video, in which he was seen distributing oxygen cylinders to those in dire need, went viral. Social media hailed him as a COVID hero, a saviour. But he was booked for flouting COVID protocols. The details of the FIR painted him as a perpetrator.

To express solidarity, I reached out to the reporter. His brother greeted me on the phone and said the administration had withdrawn the FIR, but he was too weary to speak on the matter anymore.

I didn't want to become the story in these tumultuous times, so I reminded myself to rely solely on the official reports sent to the state headquarters and not on the rumour mill that WhatsApp groups often became.

After returning to Varanasi, I sought a meeting with the district magistrate, Kaushal Raj Sharma, once more, but failed again.

I also messaged Arvind Kumar Sharma, one of PM Modi's long-time aides. In 2021, following his resignation as joint secretary, he assumed office as a BJP MLC in UP. The PMO sent him to Varanasi on 13 April to supervise the state government's COVID response.[2]

In UP, he was referred to as 'Team Delhi'. He was seen as the PM's man by Varanasi administration. This put him in direct (or indirect) contention with 'Team Yogi'.

Kaushal Raj Sharma, Varanasi's Collector, was in the PM's good books. He had been leading the district since 2019 when the Modi 2.0 regime began.

A.K. Sharma declined my request for a meeting.

As soon as he arrived in Varanasi, he had been holding video conferences with the district magistrate, divisional commissioner, superintendent of police, chief medical officer, deputy collectors, municipal commissioner and medical superintendent, among others. An MLC summoning the district's top officials to take stock of the situation, despite it not being his jurisdiction or within his purview, was bound to ruffle feathers. But given Sharma's proximity to the PM, no one was in a position to object.

A.K. Sharma was credited for establishing a 24×7 Kashi COVID Response Centre within two weeks of his arrival. The Centre collected real-time data on the number of beds available, oxygen supply and demand and the stock of essential medicines. Sharma personally visited adjoining districts in Purvanchal and other COVID hotspots to boost the morale of frontline workers.

Sharma's strategies were presented as 'innovative' in the press, but I found them to be aligned with practices already being followed in all major districts in India. COVID Command Centres everywhere were actively monitoring real-time data on healthcare resources.

Not one official wanted to comment on Sharma's style of working on record. In off-the-record conversations, they dismissed the disproportionate media coverage he got.

By the end of May, as in the rest of the country, Varanasi too began to witness a decrease in its caseload.

Team Yogi kept a close watch on A.K. Sharma's activities.

Before leaving Varanasi, I stood outside the collector's residence, chatting with the security personnel deployed at the gate, hoping to convince the collector to give me an appointment. But after waiting for an hour, I received his message declining the meeting. Kaushal Raj Sharma was among the longest serving collectors in Varanasi, from 2019 to 2022, when he was promoted to the role of divisional commissioner. In May 2025, he was deputed to Delhi under the AGMUT cadre, following the Centre's approval of his inter-cadre transfer from Uttar Pradesh for a three-year term.

There were speculations brewing within bureaucratic circles in UP that his proximity to the Prime Minister's Office (PMO) would get him a prominent post in the PMO or the national capital.

After many failed attempts at securing meetings, I started visiting the laboratories recognised as official COVID-19 testing labs by the district administration. UP was conducting 225,000–235,000 tests daily, which happened to be below the national average.

Varanasi's caseload was overwhelming for its testing labs, and the state government had imposed restrictions on most private labs, not allowing them to conduct tests. Some labs reported a deliberate reduction in testing as per the district administration's directive. Apart from the state's intervention, their operations slowed down as several of their technicians who conducted home tests contracted the virus themselves. Plus, there was a shortage of testing kits.

Among the city's major private testing facilities such as Heritage, Meridian Hospital, Oncquest, Apex, SRL and Lal Path Labs, etc., only Lal Path Labs and SRL were permitted to collect samples from homes.

Between 17 and 27 April 2021, district health records indicated that no private labs except for Lal Path Labs and SRL, carried out COVID-19 tests. Out of the thirty centres operated by Lal Path Labs in the city, merely seven were sanctioned to collect test samples.

I spoke to a Lal Path Lab worker who said that there was a scarcity of testing kits and they were advised by the authorities to limit COVID testing.

As private labs slowed down, citizens turned to the district's official testing centres. Institutions like Banaras Hindu University (BHU), the Employees' State Insurance Corporation (ESIC) and Sir Sunderlal Hospital (SSPG), in addition to Community

Health Centres (CHCs) and Primary Health Centres (PHCs), took over. When the demand for testing soared even further, the administration set up testing booths at strategic locations such as railway stations and the airport to expand coverage. Still, it wasn't enough.

With time, as resources diminished, Varanasi was testing fewer and fewer people. 4,516 RT-PCR tests were conducted on 21 April, while only 1,479 people were tested on 27 April. Despite this, the number of positive cases escalated from 1,637 on 20 April to 1,752 on 27 April.

People were desperate to get tested, but their efforts were thwarted by infrastructural bottlenecks; the waiting time grew long. The entire process, from the test to the results, was now taking nearly a week.

Dr S.S. Kannojiya, the assistant chief medical officer (ACMO) of Varanasi, refuted the claims that the private labs had been instructed to reduce their rate of testing. But he did admit that the facilities were overwhelmed by the surging demand for tests.

'The rural areas are particularly hit by the lack of resources, but we are actively enhancing our testing capabilities.' He also highlighted that the administration had ordered forty new RT-PCR machines, expected to arrive by 10 May 2021.

Contrary to the ACMO's statements, my sources within the state health department, divulged that there was, in fact, a dearth of testing kits.

'We're currently grappling with a shortage of kits, and a significant number of our lab technicians have tested positive. Our resources are stretched thin,' an official had admitted.

Between 21 April and 27 April 2021, Uttar Pradesh ranked among the ten most affected states. The data, extracted from the Covid19India.org dashboard, showed that it was recording a daily average of 34,813 new cases with an average positivity rate of 16.7 per cent.

UP cabinet minister and government spokesperson, Sidharth Nath Singh offered an optimistic outlook on recovery and normalcy.

But official statements were in stark contrast to the personal accounts of those who worked at the frontlines.

I interviewed Saurabh Kumar Singh, a twenty-eight–year–old lab technician in Varanasi employed by the National Health Mission. He had recently recovered from COVID and resumed his duty soon after testing negative. On 6 April 2021, the day he fell ill, he had collected fifty home samples across the city.

A technician from SRL, a prominent private lab network, said, 'Sometimes within hours of submitting their samples, the patients' health deteriorates rapidly, and then, it's a test of patience as days pass before the test results arrive.'

After I filed my last dispatch from Varanasi, it was time for Arunesh to go. He couldn't wait to see his family in Lucknow. I would miss Arunesh's company and his commentary. Babloo, my new driver, took the wheel.

10

War Rooms

At 2 p.m. on 27 April 2021, the corridors of Ballia's district hospital were echoing with cries of distress.

In the general ward, over twenty patients lay on stretchers or on the floor, unattended, not one doctor or nurse in sight. Their families were crowding around the reception and pharmacy.

The last time I was inside a COVID ward, every attendant wanted to tell their story. They would mob me so that I would record what they had to say. I had been adhering to the new normal of several layers of masks and a face shield over them. But that afternoon, I had forgotten the face shield in the car.

For ten long minutes, a man on a stretcher in the middle of the general ward remained still. He did not have a companion by his side. I asked around to find out if he had an attendant. Most people were too busy caring for their own families to pay attention to me. Did anyone even know that this man was lying there?

Like any other public hospital, here too the walls were peeling off, the floor was cracked, and a mixed, pungent smell of urine and gutka hung in the air. I settled down in a dim corner of the ward to watch and take notes. Half an hour passed but the man continued to lie there—unclaimed and unnoticed. I finally decided to walk up to him. Just then, a male nurse entered the ward and was immediately surrounded by concerned family members.

I felt compelled to draw the nurse's attention to this unattended patient. He came and checked his pulse.

'He has passed away.' And then he moved to the next patient, then the next and the next. People kept dropping dead within hours of making it to emergency wards.

'Yours'?

'87? Okay.'

'Yours?'

'60? Okay.'

'Yours?'

'50? Okay.'

The nurse was going around checking the oxygen levels of the patients scattered on the floor.

The ward had only two stretchers—one had been claimed by the dead man. His blue slippers lay beside the stretcher. His abdomen was distended, his legs dangled over the edge of the stretcher, one hand hung by his side and his mouth was open. He seemed to be in his late forties or early fifties.

I asked the staff about his relatives, but his identity remained a unknown. If he had been brought to the hospital by someone, they were nowhere to be found now.

I waited some more.

A woman walked towards me and bent down to touch my feet. I was startled. Behind her was a frazzled young man, making calls on his phone, frantically looking for help.

Forty-five–year–old Draupadi Devi's husband, and twenty-two–year–old Deepak Kumar's father, Bhoora Prasad, fifty, had an oxygen saturation of just 72.

The family's livelihood depended on Prasad's income as an e-rickshaw driver. A week ago, he had contracted a fever and cold. In these parts of Uttar Pradesh—Ballia, Ghazipur, Mirzapur, Jaunpur and Varanasi—a severe heat wave swept through May and June. So people contracting a fever was nothing out of ordinary.

'We assumed it was a heatstroke,' Deepak explained. They took him to a small clinic close to where they lived.

As members of the Gond tribe, the family lacked generational wealth. They had to work every day to put food on their plates. However, Draupadi, who had studied up to class eight, supplemented the household's earnings by stitching clothes and becoming a self-help group member. The family relied heavily on the monthly allocation of five kg of grains under the state subsidy initiative. Deepak was pursuing a three-year polytechnic course in Mathura district. Three days after being treated for a heatstroke, Bhoora Prasad's condition worsened and he started gasping for air. That's when they sent samples to test him for COVID. The results came three days later. Prasad was COVID positive.

The family rushed him to Shriji Hospital, a private nursing home run by Dr V.K. Gupta. After examining Prasad, Gupta gave two options to his son Deepak—either arrange an oxygen cylinder or find an ambulance to transfer him to a COVID hospital.

Without an ambulance or oxygen cylinder, the family managed to transport Prasad to City Hospital in an auto-rickshaw, but they were refused admission there. After multiple failed attempts at various private hospitals, they ended up at the district hospital. Dr Gupta had despatched Deepak with a grim warning: call your near and dear ones, because your father is 'half an hour's guest'; he won't last longer than that.

Deepak shared the doctor's words with his mother. Draupadi panicked and started begging other patients on oxygen support to grant her husband half an hour.

Prasad lay there with an IV line up his arm. He was too weak to sit up. A blue bag containing some medicines and a bottle of kaadha lay beside him. Draupadi kept rubbing his back to soothe him.

'Bacha leejiye humaare pati ko, aapke pair padte hain. Bacha leejiye.' (Please save my husband, I beg at your feet.) Draupadi attempted to touch my feet again.

In her desperation, she began to take off whatever little gold she was wearing, 'Take whatever you need for his treatment but please save him.'

She had mistaken me for a doctor. Before I could console her, I found myself struggling to breathe.

I ran out of the ward and sat under a tree. For a moment, everything around me ceased to make sense. I went outside to find my car, to drink some water. I also took a bottle of sanitiser and a face shield. I calmed down somewhat and re-entered the general ward. I exchanged phone numbers with Deepak, hoping to find some help for his father.

In the same ward, thirty-five–year–old Sarita Devi clung to her husband. She was lying on the floor, her SpO2 was at 40. Her family had exhausted all efforts to secure medical aid for her and returned empty-handed to the district hospital.

Nearby, another patient named Lali lay on the floor, struggling to breathe, her chest wracked with relentless pain.

Everyone in the room needed urgent medical attention. The doctor was preceded by a young man in a bloodstained shirt, his head bandaged and flanked by four men who were either making phone calls or running to the pharmacy. The injured man was not wearing a mask. The doctor, upon seeing blood on his shirt, rushed to him.

But in the next instant, he started shouting, asking the attendants to leave the hospital immediately. One of the four men took out his phone to record the doctor's outburst. Initially, the doctor seemed callous. But soon, a different picture emerged.

The doctor went around the ward, checking on the patients lying on the floor. Then he spoke again. 'Why are you sitting among COVID positive patients? Do you want to die?' he snapped at another young man sitting amidst the crowd.

The wounded man's companions were still recording the doctor.

'Go on, record me! I don't care. I will slap you.'

The doctor addressed the crowd, emphasising that the injured man wasn't suffering from Coronavirus but had been injured in a minor land dispute.

'They are fighting over land while the world grapples with death itself. They expect us to prioritise their petty conflicts over COVID patients who could die any moment,' the doctor expressed his frustration.

I was told that the injured man was the fifth to arrive under these circumstances.

Land disputes were quite common in the region. The panchayat polls, too, had ignited clashes among villagers, and these cases added to the caseload at local hospitals.

On 30 April 2021, Sajid and I visited Ghazipur district, about ninety km from Ballia.

I had lined up an interview with Dr J.C. Mourya, chief medical officer (CMO) of Ghazipur district. When I told him about Ballia's district hospital, he weighed in, 'Whenever there are local body elections, we witness an increase in such disputes. For many, it is moochh ka sawaal, a question of honour.'

During our interview, his phone kept ringing constantly, and after a point, he could no longer ignore the calls.

'Dekhiye, mahaamaari phaili hai, aap ye ladai-jhagda ghar mein suljhaaiye, emergency ward mein pair rakhne ki jagah nahi hai, yahaan patti nahin hogi.' (Look, we're all dealing with a pandemic. Resolve your fights at home. The emergency ward has no room to even set foot in, let alone attend to your injuries), he calmly advised the caller. The call was meant to do 'pairavi', or provide a reference for admission to a hospital.

Ghazipur and Ballia were swept into the political currents of panchayat polls. Since regular hospital wards were shuttered, those injured in panchayat poll clashes knocked on the doors of COVID wards.

In Dr J. Mourya's office, Sajid and I were the sixth and seventh attendees, along with five of his subordinates.

'If I were to send these five for testing, I have no doubt they'd all test positive. But I simply cannot spare anyone,' Mourya remarked.

Ghazipur and Ballia, home to 3.6 and 3.2 million people respectively, were witnessing their healthcare crumble.

The scenes in the emergency wards at the government hospitals were grim—patients gasping for breath, their families fighting for medical attention, bodies of those who didn't make it lying unattended and doctors near breaking point.

Patients came—on bikes, bullock carts, e-rickshaws—from places as far as forty km away. But the emergency wards were too small to even fit everyone in, let alone provide adequate care.

As the clock neared 3 p.m., the lone doctor attending to patients in the Ghazipur hospital general ward confided in me between hurried consultations, 'This is now a war room. The virus is attacking from all sides. We are losing our minds.'

Inside that war zone, acute chest pain and breathlessness were making it difficult for sixty-five-year-old Ramati to sit up. Her son Gunjan Paswan, shared his plight, 'I rode 25 km on a bike as her health deteriorated overnight. I had no other option. Even if she is COVID positive, we can't simply let her die.'

Every few minutes, Paswan would plead with a doctor to take a look at his mother, but the doctor was surrounded by desperate family members of other patients.

A few steps away, eighty-four–year–old Kamlapati Rai shared his oxygen with two other patients. A member of his family said they had been waiting to be examined for four hours.

'They are saying we can give you a bed in the isolation ward, but we will have to arrange oxygen for him. What use is the bed then?' he added.

This ward only had six makeshift beds, with one compounder and a doctor in attendance. Two people manned the reception desk, while about hundred people waited for treatment.

As the crowd kept growing by the hour, impatient family members started getting into fights with the staff.

'Kab see keh rahe hain ki dekh lo, mar jayenge toh dekhenge? Kisliye emergency ward likha hai? Maut ka ward likh dijiye.' (How long must we beg for attention? Will you only examine him once he's dead? This is not an emergency ward, call it a death ward), a person yelled out sheer frustration.

Outside the ward, four patients were lying in the corridor in critical condition. 'These are the unlucky ones who could not even make it to the emergency ward floor,' said someone accompanying a patient.

This was a difficult story to write. Despite the situation on the ground, the district health data revealed that Ghazipur and Ballia were testing about 2,000 and 2,832 people, respectively, daily, in April.

Dr Ashok Rai, president of the Indian Medical Association in UP criticised these numbers as insufficient for these populous Purvanchal districts.

For a population this large, the two districts had only 255 and 900 hospital beds, respectively, while they struggled with a caseload of nearly 10,000 active cases.

It took the combined efforts of a journalist, an activist, a district magistrate and even SOS calls on Twitter to change the fate of Deepak's father.

Before I left Ballia late on the evening of 27 April, I coordinated with Aditi Singh, the district magistrate, and a Twitter acquaintance. Her assistance was crucial in admitting Deepak's father to a COVID dedicated hospital. Within an hour of my call with Aditi, three ambulances arrived outside the district hospital to transport Bhoora Prasad to a dedicated COVID centre outside the city.

'When we reached the government facility, doctors were waiting to receive my father,' Deepak told me later. However, even with the Collector's direct involvement, the family could not secure a bed until ten that night. Hospital admission didn't guarantee immediate treatment. Bhoora Prasad now had oxygen support but he still needed to be examined by a doctor.

When I flagged this to Aditi the next morning, she assured me that she had assigned one of her officers to provide emergency assistance.

As a Collector, she was dealing with hundreds of such requests. She was thoroughly frustrated. A patient had assaulted a doctor, and another family had attacked a rapid response team. The administration had been dealing with such cases all day, every day. She also recounted incidents where people had requested oxygen for patients who didn't need it.

I guaranteed her that Deepak's father genuinely needed it. At times, I had to reassure Deepak and encourage him to trust the officers' efforts.

In the ward where Bhoora Prasad battled for his life, Deepak and his mother witnessed deaths every day.

'People were dying as soon as they got admitted. My father's oxygen kept dropping and picking up again.' Deepak recounted the days he spent in the ward.

He had called me after getting his father discharged. I was in Bihar at the time.

Draupadi wanted to speak to me. She called me, ma'am, to which I said that I was her daughter's age. She said, 'Uss din aapne jo kiya, aap hum sabse badi ho gayi hain.'

Over the years, I have stayed in touch with the family and they still express gratitude for their father's survival. But the toll that fortnight took on this family reflects the struggles faced by lakhs of families in India. For Prasad's treatment, the family had to borrow up to 1 lakh rupees.

'Everything was being sold at double the price. My father survived, but we have a debt ₹30,000-₹35,000,' Deepak said. Financial constraints forced Deepak to pursue a BA course in Ballia instead of his desired B. Tech degree.

His younger brother, Dheeraj Kumar, now twenty-two, also completed a polytechnic diploma. Meanwhile, Priyanka Kumari, their older sister, is trying to get a teaching job by enrolling in the BTC (Basic Teacher Certificate) course.

Prasad has resumed driving the e-rickshaw. Both Prasad and Draupadi are determined to send their sons to Allahabad, a coaching hub, to prepare for competitive exams.

'My sister's marriage is a priority for us,' Deepak told me over the phone recently. However, the path to securing a government job is as challenging as finding a bed during the second wave. Paper leaks have plagued India's recruitment system in recent times, leaving Deepak and Dheeraj with limited prospects.

11

The Deadly Panchayat Polls

I had never met Kalyani Agrahari but I felt a deep connection with her dreams and struggles. Her story resonated not just with me, but with millions of women who enter the workforce.

Kalyani, twenty-seven–year–old primary school teacher from Jaunpur district, tragically succumbed to the virus. I received a photo of her in a WhatsApp forward. The image showed her standing outside a government school, dressed in a sea-green saree, a blue shawl and red bangles on her wrists. Her eyes were bright and her smile radiated with pride. The caption revealed that she was eight months pregnant when she had contracted COVID after being forcibly assigned to poll duty during the Panchayat elections.

The reason I am telling this story lies not in her death but in the way she died.

I verified the lead by calling the phone numbers mentioned alongside the photo on the WhatsApp group. One of those numbers belonged to Kalyani's sister. When I asked her about Kalyani, I heard sobs on the other end.

'I'm sorry, but I just wanted to confirm the news about your sister being eight months pregnant while passing away on poll duty. I saw a photo…' I asked hesitantly.

'My sister is no more. Yes, she was eight months pregnant. The post is accurate,' her younger sister, Rani, confirmed through her tears.

Kalyani was the first child of Suresh Chandra Agrahari and Chandrawati Devi, born in Pawai Bazaar, a small town about twenty km from Azamgarh district.

Suresh ran a hardware shop in the local market. Kalyani had two younger brothers and a sister. Unlike many girls in the town, who often didn't have the opportunity to pursue higher education, Kalyani's family, belonging to the Baniya caste, had a tradition of educating their daughters. While they didn't send them to metro cities for courses in fashion, hospitality or technology, they ensured the girls were enrolled in local colleges.

Teaching and banking are among the most preferred professions for young women like Kalyani and her sister in rural and small-town India. This is the extent to which families are willing to educate and empower their daughters. These jobs offer three key benefits: job security, local postings and societal respect.

After completing class twelfth, Kalyani pursued her BA, B.Ed and BTC from local colleges, ticking all the right boxes for a 'good girl'. In 2018, Kalyani's family arranged her marriage to Deepak Chand from Jaunpur.

Deepak, after completing his B.tech, worked as a boiler operator in a sugar mill in Najibabad, Ghaziabad. Before their wedding in April 2018, Deepak visited Kalyani's home to meet her in person to give a nod to the proposal. Their meeting, in the presence of family members, lasted for only about ten-fifteen minutes. They exchanged names, discussed their educational backgrounds and shared their aspirations. Kalyani expressed her desire to work, and her straightforward, simple approach to life won Deepak's heart, he told me in an interview.

After the marriage, Kalyani went to live with Deepak and his family in their ancestral village, Pataila, a gram panchayat located thirty-five km from Jaunpur. In 2019, Deepak sent her to Allahabad for a short course to prepare for the government teaching exam, which she successfully cleared in May 2020. She was among the 69,000 candidates who passed the exam for assistant basic teachers in Uttar Pradesh.

However, their appointments became controversial, and the issue was taken to the Allahabad High Court and then to the Supreme Court by the Uttar Pradesh Prathmik Shiksha Mitra Association.

In November 2020, the Supreme Court ordered that the selected candidates be recruited.[1]

Finally, in January 2021, Kalyani, along with 68,599 other candidates, joined as an assistant basic teacher in UP.

It was Kalyani's first month as an assistant teacher when the country was hit by the second wave. Though on the personal front, this period was filled with joy for Kalyani and her husband as they eagerly awaited the arrival of their first child. She was eight months pregnant. When she saw her name on the list of government teachers assigned to panchayat poll duty on 15 April 2021, she became anxious.

'She didn't want to do it. In her condition, it would be a challenge to travel that far and sit in one place for long,' Deepak said.

To avoid any complications, Kalyani and Deepak travelled thirty-two km from Pataila to Jaunpur Vikas Bhavan to submit an application requesting exemption from election duty.

'I am a primary school teacher posted at Moina Composite School in Khutahan block. I have been assigned to the Panchayat polls and my code number is 24146. Due to my critical pregnancy, I will not be able to appear for the posting. Therefore, it is my humble request to the district election officer to relieve me from my duty,' she pleaded in her application to the district election officer cum district magistrate.

The trip, however, proved to be futile. She wasn't exempted from duty; instead, she was threatened that she would face an FIR and also risk losing her salary if she did not report to duty. Fifteen days later, she died in a Jaunpur hospital. Her death certificate said she was COVID positive. This was her first posting, she hadn't even received her first salary yet.

Kalyani was among the government employees (said to be over 2000 in number),[2] who contracted the virus while deployed for panchayat poll duty, which was held in four phases (on 15, 19, 26 and 29 April) for about 850,000 local body seats during the second wave. However, what transpired before her death was not just a tragedy but, according to her family, cold blooded murder.

Before the polls, election workers, including the primary teachers, were called to attend training sessions, a standard practice for all types of elections—Panchayat, State Assembly or Lok Sabha. The Uttar Pradesh Primary Teachers' Union and the Uttar Pradesh Teachers' Association wrote to the State Election Commission on 12 April, expressing their concerns, describing the second wave as 'terrifying'.[3] Despite these warnings, the state went ahead and conducted the elections.

According to the data declared by the government, over 11 lakh government employees were assigned to election duty in Panchayat polls; 65 per cent of them, over 6.5 lakh, were teachers.[4] In the last week of April, addressing the alarming situation, the UP Pradeshiya Prathamik Shiksha Sangh released a list with the names of over 700 teachers who had died of COVID since the beginning of the pandemic and requested Chief Minister Yogi Adityanath and the state election commissioner to put the counting of votes on hold.[5] The UP Shikshak Mahasangh also released a list of 577 teachers and support staff who had died after being deployed for panchayat poll duty, as reported by *India Today*.[6])

In response to the rising number of teacher deaths, the Allahabad High Court issued a show-cause notice to the Uttar Pradesh State Election Commission, demanding an explanation as to why action should not be taken against it and its officials for failing to enforce COVID-19 protocols.[7]

After nationwide outrage and criticism, in a statement to the media, the Yogi Adityanath government clarified that they did not initially want to hold the panchayat elections, it was an Allahabad High Court order that forced them to conduct it before 30 April. The state government also said that there was no proof that the teachers had died while on poll duty.[8]

Minister of State (Independent Charge) for Basic Education Satish Chandra Dwivedi said it was wrong to say that the teachers on poll duty had died of COVID-19.[9]

When the tussle between the state and the court didn't yield any results, the unions resorted to boycotting counting day on 2 May.[10] Some teachers joined the call, while others felt too powerless to rebel against the mighty state.

Kalyani had shown remarkable courage by travelling to the concerned officials to have her case heard, despite there being a risk of losing her job.

'She was anxious about not being able to sit for long periods during poll duty. We returned home disheartened from Vikas Bhavan that day. Unhone kaha nayi naukri hai, salary nahin milegi.' (They said it's a new job, you won't get a salary), Deepak said this to me days after Kalyani's death.

Kalyani attended the training exercise at the polling booth assigned to her on 14 April, the day before the polls.

'After she returned, she fell sick, and kept getting sicker and sicker. First, she complained of body ache then she came down with a fever and then she could not get up,' Deepak recounted.

'She was forced to travel 32 km to reach the polling station on 15 April. She spent more than twelve hours on the field. She was very unwell when she returned home,' Deepak remembered his wife's final days.

Kalyani passed away on 24 April at a Mahila Chikitsalay (women's hospital), just two days before their third wedding anniversary on 26 April.

Deepak showed me the last photos of his wife, lying in a semi-conscious state on oxygen support.

'I want to see our baby. Save me please,' were her last words to Deepak.

'Pehle din ki shuruaat tumse hoti thi, ab tumhari yaadon se hoti hai.' Deepak's WhatsApp status, changed on 31 May 2021, remains the same four years later. In his display picture, Deepak and Kalyani are standing by a pond with a teeka on their foreheads, and posing for a selfie. This photograph was taken when she had shared the news of her pregnancy with Deepak. Wearing an orange shawl, a nose ring and dark lipstick, she looks like someone who is eagerly looking forward to her future.

When I spoke to Deepak in April 2021, his voice was filled with rage as he struggled to come to terms with the loss of his unborn child and wife. 'The officials killed her. They should all be booked for criminal negligence.'

Kalyani's father, Suresh Chandra Agrahari, was inconsolable.

'When they knew she was eight months pregnant, they could have sent me to poll duty instead of her,' he cried over the phone.

'Maine usey itna padhaya likhaya ki kuch banegi, lekin system se kya mila? Ek maut. Meri beti ki jaan panchayat vibhag ke adhikariyon ki vajah se gayi.' (I educated her so she could achieve something in life, but what did the system give us? Death. My daughter died because of the officials in the panchayat department.)

Recalling the days after Kalyani returned from poll duty (on 15 April), the family told me that they decided to take her to a hospital on 18 April after her fever did not subside for two days.

'We approached the Akbarpur district hospital first but were turned away. We then went to Isha Hospital in Jaunpur, JP Dubey Hospital in Shahganj, Kumar Hospital in Jalalpur, Ambedkarnagar, Mayo Hospital in Jalalpur, Sunita Hospital in Jaunpur, Trauma Center in Jaunpur and Sadar Hospital in Jaunpur, one by one, but there was no bed anywhere. We ran from pillar to post for three days. Precious time was lost … After her SpO2 dropped to 40, we went for a COVID test and also arranged for an oxygen cylinder,' her father recounted.

I dialled Nitish Singh, then SDM (sub-divisional magistrate) in Jaunpur to get the official version of the sequence of events in the case of Kalyani's death, as other senior officials such as CDO (chief development officer) and Collector, were inaccessible.

'If someone is unwell, the person has to write to our medical committee. To relieve them on medical grounds is a decision taken by that committee. This incident (of Agrahari) is unfortunate, I will see if I can help the family in any way,' Nitish Singh told me.

When I was reporting on the deaths of teachers from being assigned to poll duty, many families were too scared to go on record. I contacted several families in Ballia and other districts, but most leads went cold.

When I met the families in person, they initially talked about the symptoms and the fact that their loved ones had been suspected of COVID. However, once they learned the story would be published, they backed out.

'Madam, humein khabar nahin karaani' (we would prefer not to report this), many requested, fearing harassment from the government. Out of fear, many families didn't even get COVID tests done for the deceased teachers.

Nirbhay Singh, a member of a teachers' association in Ballia district, explained, 'Many teachers who showed COVID symptoms went to block officials to get their duty cancelled, but they were threatened with FIRs and voluntary retirement.'

So I went ahead and published Kalyani's story on 30 April. It was a tough story to write. I broke down several times while working on its drafts.

Kalyani's story put the spotlight, both national and international, on the issue of teachers' deaths. There were multiple follow-ups, and I began to see many families overcome their fear and come forward to speak to the media.

What followed was nothing short of a travesty. First, the families lost their earning members to a callous system and then they had to endure a long administrative battle to get their deceased loved ones listed as COVID deaths.

After initially denying that the teachers caught COVID during poll duty, the Uttar Pradesh government responded to the criticism, by announcing that it would provide compensation to the families of the deceased teachers.

According to a report published in the *Economic Times*, the government instructed district magistrates to collect data on teachers who died after contracting COVID during panchayat poll duty. By the last week of May 2021, the district magistrates reportedly identified only three teachers who had died 'on duty'.[11]

'This is a mockery of death,' one of the families of a teacher in Ballia commented.

This figure of three starkly contrasted the Uttar Pradesh Prathmik Shiksha Sangh's claim that over 1,600 teachers and workers from the basic education department had died after contracting the virus during poll duty.[12]

The state could only identify three names because the rest of the families were not able to furnish the required documentation and meet the rules laid by the state election commission. As per the old rules, compensation was only provided if the employee died on duty or while travelling to and from the place of duty—typically within a day or two, depending on how far the employee travelled.

It took another round of protests, letter submissions and reporting to get the government to revise the compensation protocols. Now it was modified to include anyone who died within thirty days of their duty.

The Allahabad High Court monitored the case closely. Ultimately, the state government made some changes and informed the court that it would provide a compensation of thirty lakh rupees to the families of deceased teachers and shiksha mitras who died on poll duty.[13] But the court was of the opinion that thirty lakh rupees were too little.

It observed that the compensation offered to families of the teachers who died due to 'the deliberate act on the part of the State and the State Election Commission to force them to perform duties in the absence of RT-PCR support' should be at least one crore.[14]

Referring to this order, the Uttar Pradesh Prathmik Shiksha Sangh also demanded a compensation of 1 crore rupees for the families of deceased teachers.

After several months of negotiation, the compensation was finalised at thirty lakhs. Uttar Pradesh received 3,078 applications for compensation. Of those, 2,128 were found eligible by the state. Out of 2,128, 50 per cent were teachers. The state also included government workers and teachers who had tested negative for COVID-19 but died of post-COVID complications in the compensation list.[15] On 26 August 2021, UP's additional chief secretary, Manoj Kumar Singh, signed a letter instructing the State Election Commission to transfer 606 crores to the district headquarters.

The district magistrates were then directed to transfer thirty lakhs to the bank accounts of the deceased teachers' next of kin.

Deepak received his compensation within months of the announcement. However, one task remains pending to this day.

He recalls that Jaunpur's then basic shiksha adhikari, Praveen Kumar Tiwari, came to see him along with ten other subordinates after his wife's passing.

'Do a BTC or B.Ed to get a compensatory job,' Tiwari had advised him. At thirty-two, without much thought, Deepak enrolled in a private college in Mathura, spending two lakhs to get a B.Ed degree. In 2022, Deepak even cleared the CTET (Central Teacher Eligibility Test) exam.

He learnt later that the degree was useless for him. A Supreme Court verdict in August 2023 mandated that only the BTC diploma holders are eligible to apply for primary teacher posts.[16] Until then,

Deepak had hoped to secure a basic primary teacher's position on compensatory grounds.

For the three years following his wife's passing, he kept travelling to Lucknow to try and meet the principal secretary or the director general of the Basic Education Department in order to secure a compensatory job as a basic primary teacher in place of his deceased wife. He also wrote to the chief minister, requesting a relaxation in rules to allow him to get the job on compensatory grounds since his case is both rare and tragic.

He has left no stone unturned in his quest for the job. He tried to meet Basic Education Minister Sandeep Singh through his private secretary, and approached Jaunpur Vidhansabha MLA, Girish Chandra Yadav, too. Both accepted his request letters, only to forward them with a note that says, 'niyam-anusar karein' (do as per rules).

'When my pregnant wife was forced to undertake poll duty, bypassing rules, why can't the same officials give me the job? Why do they cite rules to deny me a compensatory position?' Deepak asks.

He refers to a series of tweets made by the then Minister of State (Independent Charge) for Basic Education, Satish Chandra Dwivedi, in May 2021, where Dwivedi discussed compensatory jobs for the dependents of deceased teachers.

'Earlier, dependents were recruited against Group D vacancies despite being eligible for Group C due to a lack of vacancies in the latter category. Now, these dependents will be recruited against surplus posts under Group C.'

Born in 1988, Deepak has now exceeded the age limit for BTC, which is capped at thirty-five. He is now ineligible for the basic primary teacher's position.

After being informed by the Basic Education Department about the 2023 Supreme Court verdict, he realised he would never get the job. So, he began his efforts to secure a Group D post.

The job on compensatory grounds must be claimed within five years. Having lost the chance to become a teacher, he has made peace with the idea of becoming a peon, so long as it is a government job.

'Last option chaprasi ki naukari hai. Yeh kam se kam berozgaar hone se achcha hai.' The last option is a peon's job. It is better than being unemployed,' he says.

12

Buxar: A District Without a Functional Ventilator

I, like millions of other Indians, eagerly sought vaccination. Senior journalists were advocating for journalists to be classified as frontline workers, given their exposure on the ground. As it happens, opinions were divided on this matter too. Some even argued against it.

Opinion pieces continued to call for the liberalisation of India's vaccine policy. Until the second wave hit, it was believed that only the elderly would be severely affected. It took the Indian government several months to decide that individuals above the age of eighteen also needed vaccination, as young people, too, were ending up on ventilators and oxygen beds. The line of treatment that worked for one patient did not work for another. A person with oxygen saturation below 40 would recover, while another with levels above 80 didn't survive. Even fully vaccinated doctors succumbed to the virus.

On 19 April, Prime Minister Narendra Modi held a meeting with key healthcare stakeholders, including pharmaceutical companies, doctors and cabinet ministers. Following the meeting, they announced that individuals between eighteen to forty-five years of age would also be vaccinated.[1]

The central government said that the liberalised and accelerated Phase-3 Strategy of COVID-19 vaccination would allow states, private hospitals and industrial establishments to procure vaccines directly from manufacturers. According to a notification published by the Press Information Bureau (PIB), individuals above eighteen years of age were going to be eligible for vaccination starting 1 May under the National Vaccine Strategy. Within just ten days, states had to procure vaccines for a large, eager, young population.

However, unlike frontline workers and those above forty-five, it wasn't easy for people aged eighteen–forty-five to get vaccinated. The country that once spoke of exporting vaccines now faced acute shortage at a crucial juncture. Based on the situation I witnessed on the first day of the vaccination drive in Varanasi district, it appeared that the government had no concrete plan and the announcement had been made hastily.

People were desperate to get vaccinated, but there weren't enough slots available. They first had to register on the CoWIN portal (www.cowin.gov.in), after which they would book appointment slots before going to authorised vaccination centres.

The process for states to purchase vaccines was chaotic. Manufacturers were required to supply 50 per cent of their monthly Central Drugs Laboratory (CDL) output to the central government and the remaining 50 per cent to the open market and states.[2] This meant that the states had to manage the placement and delivery of vaccines on their own. Sates, private hospitals and other establishments could place orders based on the prices declared by the manufacturers. So, the states had to pay for the vaccines from their exchequer, they weren't free for everyone.

In Uttar Pradesh, walls were plastered with large posters put up by local BJP leaders, thanking PM Modi for free vaccines.

According to a report by PTI, some states were informed by the Serum Institute of India (SII) that the delivery of consignments with the Covishield vaccine would not start before 15 May.[3] As a result, between the announcement and 1 May, most states were unable to begin vaccinating those above eighteen years of age. Reports emerged that manufacturers were not committing to timely supply of vaccines to the states.

In November 2020, Union Health Minister Harsh Vardhan announced that the government planned to vaccinate around 25–30 crore people by July–August.[4] According to a report published in *The Hindu*, India had administered 12.4 crore vaccine doses by 19 April since the vaccine drive had begun on 16 January.[5] Despite opening vaccination to individuals above forty-five years of age on 1 April, by 19 April, only 8 per cent of the population had received their first dose, and just 1 per cent had received their second one.[6]

The vaccination drive was adversely affected in April due to the deadly second wave, the ongoing farmers' agitation in states like Haryana, Punjab and western UP, and vaccine hesitancy.

At the same time, in the national capital, one of the most affected cities, CM Arvind Kejriwal requested people not to crowd vaccination centres.

He told the media, 'I request you not to queue up at vaccination centres tomorrow. As soon as vaccines come, we will make proper announcements. Only then people with appointments can start coming to the centres.' Imagine the panic, chaos and confusion on the ground. Across the country, young people were travelling hundreds of miles to get vaccinated at rural Primary Health Centres (PHCs) because the vaccination centres in the city did not have enough vaccines.[7]

When the government announced that individuals above eighteen years of age could register for vaccination on CoWin at 4 p.m. on 28 April, the app and website crashed within minutes.

On the morning of 1 May, I was in Varanasi. I sat with my laptop, ready to secure a vaccination slot. I searched for the nearest vaccination centres, but none showed empty slots. Desperate, I tried a Primary Health Center (PHC) dozens of kilometres away, but they too were fully booked. I was disheartened.

The eighteen-plus vaccination drive was launched with limited stock, and vaccines were distributed like gold. For instance, the CoWIN app listed around 110 centres, but government data indicated that only seventeen centres were functional for this age group in Varanasi.

Uttar Pradesh rolled out the vaccination drive in only seven districts: Lucknow, Kanpur, Prayagraj, Meerut, Bareilly, Varanasi and Gorakhpur.

I went to the BHU vaccine centre, followed by the Mahila Chikitsalay vaccination centre, and then the remaining centres in Varanasi.

Vaccination centres were well managed, with proper reception areas, chairs, and posters for each eligible group. Nurses and staff were clad in PPE suits, and the administration had set up tents labelled as rooms one, two and three. The purpose of this numbering was to isolate the queues and provide privacy and space, unlike other vaccination settings where transmission doesn't occur through touch or sneezing. This setup was to maintain physical distance.

Health officials at the Covid Command Centre admitted that within a minute of the vaccine becoming available online, slots ran out.

An official at the BHU centre said, 'Now that both age groups are coming in huge numbers, we have to turn them away due to limited stock.'

At Mahila Chikitsalay (women's hospital), an official at the registration desk said, 'People are coming in unprecedented numbers.' Even as he spoke, nearly seventy people were waiting in queue.

At the BHU centre, I met Varun Kumar, a young man in his late twenties. Like me, he had been trying to register online but couldn't secure a slot. So he rushed to the BHU centre without an appointment. 'There was some glitch on the website, so I came to the centre. There is panic all around. It is better to get vaccinated as soon as possible. But I am told they have limited stock for us.' Varun hoped that if someone didn't show up, he might get their vaccine.

Can you guess how many people aged eighteen to forty-five were vaccinated in India on 1 May? Only 86,023. And only eleven states managed to procure vaccines for this age group.[8]

Without having received the life-saving jab, Sajid and I moved on to Buxar on 2 May. The first things we needed were food and accommodation. Although Bihar had announced a full-fledged lockdown, the extent of restriction varied from district to district, depending on the district magistrate. Buxar allowed shops to stay open until 1 p.m., but we arrived after that and found everything closed.

Uttar Pradesh was already under a weekend lockdown and night curfews, but Nitish Kumar was hesitant to impose a complete lockdown remembering its impact on the poor in 2020. Whenever a district magistrate suggested a complete lockdown during their video conference with the CM, Nitish Kumar would dismiss the idea.

A government source told me that he was reluctant because a complete lockdown would hit the poor the hardest. They were already out of jobs.

A civil servant based in Patna, who was a part of CM Nitish Kumar's video conferences, commented, 'He is a bit reluctant about the lockdown. He keeps emphasising how the poor have already suffered during the first wave. If we impose a strict lockdown again, there will be thousands facing starvation.'

However, as the number of cases began to rise, Nitish Kumar felt compelled to announce a total lockdown on 15 May.

Bihar's opposition leader, Tejashwi Yadav took to Twitter to criticise Nitish Kumar for failing to enforce the lockdown earlier: 'For the last fifteen days, the entire opposition has been demanding a lockdown, but "Chhote Sahab" was following the orders of "Bade Sahab" that there can't be a lockdown till 2 May. Now, when the disease has spread from village to village, they have started this pretence. Stop this low-level gimmick and politics in this crisis.' Politics aside, the lockdown in Bihar, initially set to end on 15 May, was extended for several months.[9]

We reached on a Sunday. Buxar city wore a deserted look. The only decent hotel in Buxar, Vaishnavi Clark, was hosting a wedding that day. Over fifty people were scattered across the parking lot, lobby and rooms. Sajid and I had second thoughts about checking in. My Varanasi hotel also hosted weddings daily. While the government had permitted only fifty guests, these weddings had at least over a hundred attendees. During one Bengali wedding, which easily had more than fifty guests, the staff was scared to even serve them meals. There were reports from UP and Bihar of entire families getting infected. Even at the peak of the pandemic, some families went ahead with such events that often ended in disasters. In many parts of India, there were reports of grooms or brides dying within a few days of their wedding. Photos of newlyweds in PPEs went viral on social media. When we talked to the families, they often said that they'd already had to postpone the weddings for over a year and a half due to the pandemic.

We decided against staying at the hotel. Fortunately, the circuit house was vacant since no ministers or local leaders were stepping out of their homes. But the cook and other staff were unavailable. We were on our own. We went to the market, looking for small, hidden gumatis, where we could at least buy milk and have tea.

The circuit house was situated at Purana Qila, with the Ganga flowing on one side. Near the walls lived the Dom and Mushara communities. There was a temple on the banks of the Ganga. After visiting the hospital and nearby areas that day, I went to sit at the temple. It felt good to have a moment to myself as I watched the river flow. I felt like crying. This was the loneliest I had ever felt. Every single day in the last month and a half had been spent on the road, each stop a new place, yet all I had encountered was death and despair. The memory of sitting by the river that day remains etched in my mind. After dusk, I returned to the circuit house. On 3 May, as I walked through the district hospital corridors again, I struggled to find ways to tell Bihar's story.

Although Uttar Pradesh and Bihar are often mentioned together in casual conversations, their problems and the temperament of their people are noticeably different. One key difference is the way the two states run their district administrations. For instance, in Bihar, the collectors and the SPs—the ears of the state, were more willing to meet with journalists, share insights and provide data, whereas in Uttar Pradesh, I faced a lot of resistance. But when it came to the lower ranks of the district administration, there was a certain similarity. It was initially marked by hostility, which gradually softened after a few conversations. In Buxar, when I travelled to the COVID Care Centre in Civil Lines, the policemen guarding its gates did not allow me inside the COVID hospital. But when I requested District Magistrate Aman Samir's permission, he sent one of his officers, Deepak Kumar, the additional sub-divisional magistrate (ASDM), to brief me on the situation. I requested the ASDM and the policemen to allow me to go inside wearing a PPE suit, but they were adamant that no one except medical and other hospital staff was allowed. With no other option, I decided to stand outside the facility for hours and observe. As I chatted with Kumar and the police officials, I shared how I had been on the ground for more than three weeks. The more I talked about the human cost of the tragedy, the more they opened up. Within an hour, the hostility was gone and they began discussing the real situation on the ground.

Around 4 p.m., a speeding car stopped at the gate of the COVID Care Centre. The police personnel on duty asked the family emerging from it a few questions and called for a stretcher. As the four worried family members tried to rush inside, a policeman remarked, 'There's no point in hurrying now. The patient looks like a dead man.'

Unfortunately, the policeman was right.

The patient, seventy-year-old Veerendra Tiwary, was declared dead. His hospital admission was delayed because his family tried to treat him at home and when things got serious, they couldn't find a bed or an ambulance. In the end, they had to stuff him into a car and rush him to the hospital. The hospital would blame families for the delay, the families would blame the hospital and the cycle would continue. This was a common story. Buxar was declared 'Covid-free' after the 'last case' was recorded on 17 January 2021, Deepak Kumar told me as we stood outside the hospital building, surrounded by policemen and attendants.

Some distance away, a tent had been set up for families that had travelled hundreds of kilometres with their sick relatives. These families had gas stoves, tea boxes and grains with them. They cooked meals there, slept on the ground, bathed at hand pumps and relieved themselves in the open. Nearby, their clothes were hung out on wires to dry.

A 1,000 kilometres away, at AIIMS in Delhi, hundreds of families from eastern UP and Bihar lived in similar conditions for months as they could only afford the cost of treatment, not accommodation. While some complained about the heat, many had become used to it.

The COVID Care Centre, where critical patients were brought, had sixty-seven oxygen beds and had reported four to five deaths every day for the past week.

'Those who are critical do not survive,' said the ASDM of Buxar district.

A COVID-free district at the beginning of the year—between 17 January and 19 March, the district did not report any new cases.

And then, after its first case in two months on 19 March, Buxar reported twenty-three cases on 1 April. By 15 April, this number grew to a hundred per day and continued to rise.

But what went wrong? 'Around Holi, we saw a massive influx of migrants returning home. As many as twenty-three trains stop at the Buxar railway station,' District Magistrate Aman Samir explained.

Despite the administration's claim that they continued testing even after declaring the district COVID-free, the testing numbers were not really encouraging.

'We conducted 4,000 tests every day earlier. But now the number of tests has been reduced to 2,000 people every day, out of which 750 are RT-PCR and the rest are antigen,' Aman added.

A senior official in the administration, who wished to remain anonymous, told me that RT-PCR samples had to be sent to Patna, where the labs were already working beyond capacity.

On 3 May, according to figures released by the Bihar health ministry, Buxar reported 104 new COVID cases and twenty-five deaths.[10] While district officials claimed there was no shortage of oxygen, doctors and medical staff said the deaths were mainly due to lack of ventilators in government hospitals.

Buxar had only six ventilators between its two government hospitals designated for COVID treatment, and none were operational. Six dysfunctional ventilators for a population of more than 17 lakh.

'There is no functional ventilator in our district. Doctors cannot save extremely critical patients. Each day, we witness such deaths. Now I can tell just by looking at a patient whether they will survive or not,' said the policeman I was talking to. Sadar Hospital had received four ventilators from the PM CARES fund in 2020, but they were locked away on the second floor. Why? Because there was not a single person in the district who could operate these life-saving machines.

'We received them last year. But without any expert or anesthetist, we cannot operate them,' Dr Bhupendra Nath told me.

Four private hospitals in the district had six ventilators between them; none of them was functioning.

District Magistrate Aman Samir told me, 'I have held meetings with private hospitals. We are outsourcing technicians who can help us run these ventilators. Within a week, all the ventilators will be functional.'

Ventilators remained locked away across districts in Bihar.

On 3 May, Bihar reported a total of 107,667 active cases. 1,458 of them were reported from Buxar. The district administration's biggest challenge was finding a pulmonologist to operate ventilators. Until the first week of June, while I stayed in Bihar, I did not hear from any of the districts I reported on that they had found a specialist.

I also visited VK Global Hospital, a private COVID facility, still under construction, in Buxar town. The noise of construction intensified the agony of patients.

The hospital had twenty oxygen beds, charging patients 150 rupees per hour for oxygen. The staff at this hospital said that an alarming number of patients tested negative for COVID-19 but their CT scans showed symptoms. Many such patients were dying, though these deaths did not make it to the official COVID death statistics.

Buxar, the Lok Sabha constituency represented by then Union Minister of State for Health and Family Welfare, Ashwini Kumar Chaubey, did not have a medical college. Even before the pandemic, the district relied heavily on Varanasi and Patna for surgeries and emergencies requiring ventilator support. Despite multiple attempts to contact Chaubey through his PA, I could not reach him. I then reached out to the local Congress MLA Munna Tiwari for a comment. His office informed me that he would be available later in the day, but I never heard back.

Hospitals were short of medical staff as well. Dr V.K. Singh, owner of VK Global Hospital, expressed his frustration at many nurses refusing to report to duty. He said that the hospital was operating with just 'four doctors and four nurses.'

The nurses were scared for their lives.

Sadar Hospital, which could accommodate over twenty patients on oxygen support, had thirty-four sanctioned posts for doctors and sixty-three for nurses. However, as of 3 May, only twenty-four doctors and forty-six nurses were on duty, managing three times the number of patients they were equipped for.

The COVID Care Centre in Civil Lines had sixteen doctors and twenty nurses. Most doctors and staff I spoke with on the phone described this number as 'highly inadequate'.

'All these patients on oxygen support have tested negative but continue to show symptoms. We have enough oxygen but not enough equipment,' said Dr. Bhupendra Nath of Sadar Hospital. 'Also, we tried everywhere, but there is not a single oxygen flow meter available in Bihar.'

Basic medicines like paracetamol were also out of stock in some places. At Sadar Hospital, I met social activist Ramji Singh, who had come to hand over five oxygen flow meters to the facility.

The administration couldn't find a technician to run ventilators, hospitals couldn't find flow meters (equipment attached to oxygen cylinders to monitor pressure), and citizens couldn't find their elected MP, Ashwini Kumar Chaubey, who also happened to be the union minister of State for Health and Family Welfare.

Since the MP, MLAs and administration were unable to arrange a flow meter for the government hospital, Ramji Singh stepped in and managed to procure some flow meters from Meerut in Uttar Pradesh.

Despite having recently recovered from COVID-19, Ramji Singh began touring hospitals. I had first met him during my assignment on the migrant exodus in the first wave.

Ramji Singh had cultivated an image of a young, ambitious social activist and politician. His height, strong build and oratory skills worked in his favour as a political alternate. He shared his experience of working with mainstream politicians as a foot soldier for years but claimed that he became disillusioned with the conventional caste-based politics of Bihar. This led him, in his early thirties, to focus on health as a critical election issue. The Buxar district had only a handful of ambulances. He quickly stepped in to fill the gap. He hired a few private ambulances to help the needy and became active on social media. He also unsuccessfully contested the 2020 Bihar assembly polls.

In 2020, he arranged a langar (community kitchen) and other medical facilities for migrants. During the second wave, his ambulance service transported the deceased to cremation grounds.

When the Sadar Hospital administration admitted that the drivers who transported the bodies got infected with the virus, Ramji Singh came to the rescue. This was his moment to seize, after all the hard pitching he had been doing over the years. He not only voluntarily provided his vehicles to the hospital but also drove an ambulance himself when his driver fell sick.

While leaving the Sadar Hospital premises, we spotted the body of sixty-two–year–old Praduman Pal from Kodhi village lying unattended on a stretcher.

'He was gasping. We did an antigen test. The result came in half an hour, but he was already dead by then,' a nurse who had just finished her shift told me. The antigen test confirmed he was COVID positive. The body remained on the stretcher because the ambulance drivers were also sick. The patient's brother was nearby, overcome with grief and unsure how to take the body for cremation. I left Ramji with the patient's brother and left for Patna.

13

'Jo Hospital Jayega Woh Maara Jayega'

In New Delhi, finding a hospital bed in the first two weeks of May was nearly impossible. Bihar was facing a different kind of crisis during this time. The number of active cases started to decline in government hospitals. Conflicts between hospital staff and attendants became common in various parts of the state.

In rural districts, fewer patients went to COVID-dedicated wards as citizens had lost faith in the system.

To tell the story of this growing distrust between the people and the healthcare system, I spent three days at Patna's largest COVID hospitals—Nalanda Medical College & Hospital (NMCH) and Patna Medical College and Hospital (PMCH).

NMCH was established in 1970 as a private institution by Dr Vijay Narayan Singh, Dr Madhusudan Das, Dr Shailendra Kumar Sinha and Shri Krishna Kant Singh, the former Education Minister of Bihar, with a batch of 150 students. Later, it was taken over by the Government of Bihar in 1978.

Today, it is one of the key public healthcare institutions in Bihar, spanning a 100 acres and divided into two campuses. With 750 regular beds and 200 emergency beds, the hospital serves approximately 2,000 patients daily in its outpatient department (OPD).

Established as Temple Medical School in 1874, it was renamed Prince of Wales Medical College in 1925 and later became Patna Medical College and Hospital (PMCH). It is one of the oldest medical institutions in India.

With over 1,748 beds, PMCH underwent a significant expansion under the Nitish Kumar government. He laid the foundation in February 2021, allocating a budget of ₹5,540 crore, and claimed to make PMCH one of the largest hospitals in the world.[1] This new avatar, which would include a special helipad for emergency air ambulances, sixty modular operation theatres and 5,462 beds, was supposed to be completed within five years.

A decade of planning went into this redevelopment project, considered to be one of Nitish Kumar's most ambitious initiatives. Chief Minister Nitish Kumar inaugurated the new twin towers with 1,117 beds in May 2025, months before the upcoming 2025 assembly elections. The new deadline for the completion of the project has been set for March 2027.

When I visited PMCH in May 2021, the redevelopment had just begun.

'Jo hospital jayega wo mara jayega' (Whoever goes to the hospital will be killed), was the sentiment expressed by twenty-eight-year-old Munna Yadav, standing outside the COVID ward on 6 May. He was grieving and anxious as he called his family to inform them of his father, Deena Rai's death. Munna kept wiping his tears with a gamchha, as he made calls to friends and family. But with each call, his doubts about the cause of his father's death grew.

'Dead kar gaye hain. Kidney nikaal leb, dekhe ke padi. (They've declared him dead. They might remove his kidneys, we'll have to check),' he said over the phone.

When I shared this with my friends from Bihar, none could provide a clear explanation. Some believed that due to lack of adequate medical facilities, people were more susceptible to believing rumours that hospitals were trafficking the organs of COVID patients.

'I will have to check if they took out some part, stole his kidney. What if they (the doctors at the hospital) killed my father?' he told me.

Munna was one of the many attendants waiting outside the COVID ward at PMCH. About half an hour before we spoke at length, I had seen him arguing with the ward in-charge, demanding an update on his father's health and oxygen levels.

Even after he was told that his SpO2 was normal, Munna seemed ill at ease. He approached the cleaning staff to check on his father for him, and a small bribe—a fifty-rupee note—exchanged hands. But when he got no help, he approached me.

'Aap media se hain? Dikhaiye na ki koi intezam nahin hai yahaan. Pitaji bharti karaaye the lekin pata nahin kya chal raha hai.' (Are you from the media? Please show that there are no proper arrangements here. My father was admitted, but we have no updates.)

I went live for a show on our YouTube channel for about twenty to twenty-five minutes, and by the time I wrapped up, five attendants had already gathered around me, eager to share their frustrations.

There were three screens outside the ward, intended to facilitate communication between patients and their families, as attendants were strictly prohibited from entering once the patient was admitted. Only cleaning and medical staff were allowed inside. However, the screens, did not work.

Munna complained about this too and then pointed at the large rats roaming the hospital.

The air was thick with the stench of urine. Garbage was piled up in many places and dirty water from the toilets had overflowed into the corridors. Families of patients waited amidst this squalor, often paying staff members to bring water or life-saving medicines for their loved ones.

The scenes at both the government-run COVID hospitals in Patna—PMCH and NMCH—were more or less the same and, to put it mildly, bleak.

At NMCH, attendants brought their own table fans and lay down in the corridors, and while PMCH had implemented measures to prevent family members from entering the COVID ward to curb the spread of infection, NMCH had no such restrictions.

Ironically, the NMCH administration had barricaded the COVID ward and deployed security guards, but inside, families were often left to care for their own. Only two nurses oversaw fifty critically ill patients. When I visited their chamber, they were so overwhelmed with paperwork and data updates that they refused to even share their names.

Consequently, some patients were left to perform proning exercises on their own in order to breathe better, while their attendants washed clothes in the toilets or ate meals as they kept watch, disregarding their own safety.

I managed to enter the ward, wearing a helmet, with Amitesh Kumar, a man in his forties who urgently needed an ICU bed for his ailing mother. I had seen him, pacing anxiously in the parking area. His gloves had yellowed and sweat poured from his helmet—his substitute for a face shield. Amitesh's mother needed a ventilator bed. He suggested I accompany him into the COVID ward to report on the situation.

With his help, I was able to sneak in and capture photos.

Outside PMCH, an inconsolable Munna continued his tirade.

'Gaon gaon mein baat fail gayi hai, jo hospital jayega woh mara jayega.' (Every village now believes that whoever goes to the hospital will die.)

Munna tried his best to see his father while he was still alive but received no help. In anger, he threw his father's slippers into a bin, muttering, 'Poora aadmi khaa gaye, jooton ka kya karenge?' (The man is gone, what will we do with his shoes?).

Meanwhile, the families of two COVID patients admitted to PMCH pleaded with the administration for their release.

While people were willing to offer gold, property and money to secure a hospital bed, these two families wanted to vacate the beds.

'There is complete medical negligence here. The cleaning staff, who have no knowledge of checking pulse, monitoring oxygen levels, or administering medicines, are looking after the patients,' someone yelled.

It was true. Distressed families were bribing the cleaning staff to look after patients while they waited outside with makeshift living arrangements for days.

The non-functional audio-visual TV screens were installed only after families complained about not being able to see their loved ones who would die any minute now.

An official at the hospital said the system was discontinued because displaying names and other details 'amounted to an infringement of the patient's privacy'.

This outraged the attendants.

'You won't let us see our dying loved ones in person, and now you won't even allow us to see them on the screen. So, we only get to see their dead bodies wrapped in a polythene bag in the end,' an angry attendant told me.

'Doctors and nurses are nowhere to be seen. It's better if our patient dies at home than suffers this. At least that way, we will be able to see their face one last time.'

Fifty-four–year–old Reeta Devi, a resident of Gopalganj, was initially admitted to a private hospital in her district. However, her son hoped for better treatment at PMCH and managed to get her admitted there on 7 May. Just a day later, he took her home as I stood there, as she appeared to have only a few hours left to live.

'I could hear her sobs over the phone. No one was attending to her or even feeding her. Woh andar tadap rahi hai, aur main baahar. (She is suffering inside the ward, and I suffer outside). I will take her to another hospital.' Her son told me that he had sent a phone through a ward boy to hear his mother's voice.

'Dead body le jaane se accha hai, zinda wapis le jayein. Kam se kam pariwar ke beech to mare. Ye COVID ward jail jaisa hai, andar le jakar band kar diya ja raha hai. Agar wo andar mar jayengi, toh baahar hum bhi mar jayenge,' he broke down. (It is better to take her home alive than receive her dead body. At least she will die surrounded by her loved ones. This COVID ward is like a jail. They take patients in and then lock them up. If she dies inside the ward, I will also die.)

Outside the COVID ward at NMCH on 7 May, Amitesh held his phone to his ear, listening to the heartbreaking cries of his fifty-six-year-old mother, Sheela Kumari, who was admitted inside.

Sheela Kumari had tested positive on 28 April. Amitesh told me that her condition became so critical that she was turned away from seven private hospitals before finally being referred to NMCH. He said he was forced to bring her to the government facility, and not without trepidation.

'I drove her 80 km in this critical condition. But seeing the situation here, I don't know if she will survive. We are desperately searching for doctors and nurses, but there is no one. Each patient in this COVID ward has become aatm nirbhar (self-reliant). We have to arrange for oxygen, medicines and other essentials ourselves,' he said.

When I saw Sheela Devi, she was indeed gasping for her final few breaths. I accompanied him to the ventilator facility's reception, just a few metres away from the COVID ward. While my intention was to help him rather than cover his story, I also felt the need to document this on my phone. When I took it out to record the receptionist's response, it upset one of the security guards. They worried that videos of this mismanagement could cost them their jobs. I apologised and left the premises.

My coverage remained confined to writing. I captured very few videos. I encountered extremely sensitive scenes and moments on the ground, I wasn't sure how ethical it would be to expose vulnerable people to that extent. Yet I had to tell their stories and make them count. So, I managed to take some photographs capturing the shocking scenes playing out inside the wards.

This reminds me of a message actor Gajraj Rao sent me on Twitter when my reports went viral. He mentioned that he couldn't find my stories on YouTube and requested that I send him the links so he could watch them. When I explained that I was travelling solo and didn't have any video camera personnel with me, he strongly suggested that I record my experiences and compile them into a larger story once my reporting was done.

He was right.

Many people in the hospitals wouldn't initially realise I was a journalist. I had to explain myself to attendants and staff to get information. My approach to reporting wasn't intrusive; the attendants wanted to open up when they saw me taking notes in my diary.

TV reporting in the past, especially during tragedies like the Gorakhpur encephalitis outbreak, has often been labelled as insensitive and voyeuristic. But as a digital journalist without a microphone or a big camera, my approach was different. I focused on consoling people, earning their trust and listening to them. The doctors and administration were too overworked to even catch a breath.

This brings me to an important quote from the then Bihar health secretary, Pratyaya Amrit , who is now serving as the state's chief secretary. I called him more than a dozen times. He finally called me back after three days, only to say, 'Mere paas saans lene ka bhi time nahin hai (I don't even have the time to breathe). I am sorry I cannot answer any questions.'

My editors carried this quote in my story.

Throughout this assignment, family after family not only opened up about their travails but also helped me gain access to the wards.

In hospitals where the administration was hostile, such as AIIMS Patna, BHU and other hospitals in Lucknow, and did not want the media to anywhere near them, attendants were kind enough to click pictures and record videos from inside the wards and send to me on WhatsApp.

At every hospital I visited, I shared my number with dozens of families who later called me to share insights or update me about their patients.

This was excellent citizen journalism. Many viral photos that journalists from various states and districts were tweeting were initially captured by ordinary citizens.

Mobile journalism, also called MOJO, is often criticised for undermining traditional journalistic pursuits. But during the second wave and the migrant exodus, the pictures and videos captured by ordinary citizens helped corroborate the reports of many journalists on the ground.

I returned to my hotel after a long, exhausting day, but my search for a ventilator bed for Amitesh's mother continued. In the evening, I called Amitesh to check on him. He asked me to stop looking for help, his mother no longer needed it. She had passed away.

The next day, I set out for the hospitals again. Having witnessed people's distrust during my previous visits, I wanted to gather more information. So, I waited outside the mortuary at PMCH one more time. Many of the families and attendants I had met the day before were no longer there. Their patients had died, and they had left to cremate the bodies. Other distressed faces had replaced them.

That evening, I witnessed a scene where a family fought with the doctors outside the mortuary and threatened to file an FIR against the hospital. This was becoming all too common at PMCH.

The previous day, while I was waiting outside the same mortuary with Munna Yadav, another family had received the news that their grandfather, Rajeshwar Sinha, had succumbed to the virus. Rajeshwar, in his eighties, had bruises on his head.

His grandson, Debashish, took numerous photos of the bruises and demanded that the body be unwrapped.

The guards, the police and the mortuary staff struggled to manage the situation, prompting the nodal officer to be called in. Amidst the chaos, a YouTube reporter arrived and began recording on his phone, shoving it in the doctor's face. The doctor, visibly angry, told him to stop.

The confrontation lasted an hour, with the women of the family refusing to leave the mortuary. Debashish rushed to the nearby police station to file a complaint, alleging that his grandfather had been mistreated by the doctors. The family claimed that when they admitted their grandfather, there were no bruises on his forehead, the hospital staff must have mishandled him.

As the family continued to argue with the doctors and mortuary staff, a gang of stray dogs started barking on the premises. Munna was losing his patience as his father's body was next in line for the COVID crematorium, but the Sinha family refused to budge.

The doctor stood in a corner. I approached him to hear his side of the story. He explained that Sinha was an old man with some mental health issues. He had been moving from one bed to another and likely fell.

The next day, around 4 p.m., the body of seventy-one–year–old, Bhagwat Rai also arrived, wrapped in a polythene bag. As his four sons mourned his death, they took out their mobile phones to click his last photos. They were inconsolable.

Like Sinha's family and Munna Yadav, they too requested to unwrap the body to ensure that their father's kidneys and eyes had not been stolen.

Bhagwat Rai's wife, Lakhi Devi, had passed away on 24 April, also from COVID.

Before the body could be moved to the ambulance, a mortuary staff member approached one of the family members and whispered something, making him angry.

The mortuary staffer had demanded money for packing the body. The family refused to pay and shamed the staff for extorting money from a family that had just lost a loved one.

The staffer explained that he was a contractual employee and had not received his salary for the last six months.

'Salary nahi mil rahi hai. Is waqt koi aadmi dead body nahi chhoo raha hai. Daaru peekar sote hain raat ko ki neend aa jaye. Din mein pariwaaron ke sath jhagda hota hai. Hum thoda bahut maang rahe hain apne pet ke liye.' (We are not getting our salaries. No one is willing to touch a dead body at this time. We drink at night to be able to sleep. During the day, we argue with families. We are only asking for a little money to feed ourselves.)

After some time, one of the sons handed 200 rupees to the mortuary staffer and left in the ambulance.

Both government hospitals were reporting more than fifteen COVID deaths daily on an average.

Patna district had the highest number of patients in Bihar at the time, yet the two biggest government hospitals still had vacant beds. This raised the question: why were people avoiding these top government facilities? Officials noted that people were even vacating ICU beds.

According to the state health bulletin, Patna reported 1,646 new cases on 9 May, making it the district with the highest number of cases in Bihar. On the same day, the state recorded 11,259 new cases. By 8 May, the city had more than 22,000 active cases, accounting for 20 per cent of the state's total.[2])

Healthcare officials I spoke to said this was a worrying trend, because it meant people were not seeking treatment even when ill.

'This indicates a complete loss of faith in the healthcare system,' a health official at PMCH, requesting anonymity, said.

The unfounded fear that patients' organs would be stolen was also prevalent.

'Every day, families force us to uncover the bodies of COVID victims to check if their eyes and kidneys are intact. It's a nightmare for the families and for us,' said one of the PMCH officers.

The sentiment of 'better to die at home' was becoming all too common among the people of Bihar.

'But if we talk about the lack of trust in the medical fraternity, that sentiment extends even to Patna AIIMS and other hospitals here,' he told me.

After dispatching this story to Delhi, I went to a crematorium around 8 p.m. to follow up on the story of the Doms. Babloo, my driver, waited in the lanes as I took my phone and diary to Gulabi Ghat, a cremation ground for COVID-19 victims.

Four bodies were being cremated. The flames from the pyres at night, rising against the backdrop of the Ganga, looked like a scene out of the film *Masaan*. Three more bodies waited their turn.

I searched for the Doms. One of them was ready to talk, but a few others gathered around. Another, who seemed drunk, shouted that I didn't have a mic and didn't look like I was from the media.

'Koi college ki ladki lagti hai. Media se nahin.' (She looks like a college girl, not from the media.)

'We don't want to tell you anything,' his voice grew louder.

I began to feel unsafe and so left immediately.

At the entrance, the inspector of the ghat introduced himself as Vinod Kumar. He was noting down numbers on a piece of paper. He offered me a chair next to him and shared the numbers he had recorded.

On 8 May, sixty-four bodies were cremated here, thirty-three of which were COVID-19 victims. On 7 May, the number was fifty-three, with thirty-four being COVID-19 victims. On 2 May, the number was seventy-one, with thirty-eight being COVID-19 victims.

Vinod Kumar continued to call me even a fortnight later, just to share data from the cremation ghat.

When I returned to my hotel that night, I called Sajid and told him what had happened with the Doms. The next day, Sajid accompanied me to Baans Ghat.

The Doms were cooperative, and the other staff equally helpful, sharing data with me.

One of the Doms mentioned that the bodies were still coming in large numbers. Since he urgently needed to cremate a body, we left him to focus on his work. He connected me with two young boys whom he called his nephews. They lived half a kilometre away from the ghat.

'I want to see your locality,' I asked them to take us where they lived. The boys were more than happy to give us a tour. However, they feared the police might confiscate their scooter due to the strict lockdown.

When the police stopped us, I showed them my ID card and explained that the boys were helping me with a story. They allowed us to pass.

One of the boys was sixteen, amusingly named 'Shortcut'. And the other, Maharaja, was fifteen (names changed to protect identity). They worked the night shift at Baans Ghat.

'Din mein bade log kaam karte hain, raat ko laash hum dono jalaate hain,' they said. (The elders work during the day, while we burn the bodies at night.) They had a phone to watch videos on while waiting for the bodies to burn.

I asked Shortcut about his name.

'Pata nahin kisne rakh diya,' he giggled. (No idea who named me so.)

The basti where they lived was a makeshift arrangement. The kutcha houses were made of tin sheets. Shortcut and Maharaja were covering for another Dom who had fallen sick after working at Baans Ghat for twenty-four hours without a break.

Inside his one-room tenement, the sick man lay on a cot. His wife and four children stood by.

His wife complained, 'Itna laash jalaya hai, hath mein dard ho raha hai. Kapda baandh kar rakha hai.' (He has burned so many bodies that his arms hurt; he has tied cloth around them for support.)

As Shortcut and Maharaja hurried back to the ghat, we followed them. After safely dropping them off and thanking them, Sajid and I went looking for food. Interestingly, we found a McDonald's in Gandhi Maidan, but due to lockdown, they were only accepting online orders and wouldn't let us sit there and eat. So, we ordered through an app, met the delivery guy just outside the restaurant, and ate in our car.

14

Quacks in Rural Bihar

While I reported that fewer people were going to Patna's top COVID hospitals, I also needed to understand the situation in rural Bihar. Who was treating the patients in villages?

To investigate this, Sajid and I travelled together to Arrah (Bhojpur) district on 8 May. In various blocks, clinics were closed, leaving patients to fend for themselves. Abandoned by the system, patients were left in the care of pharmacists or village quacks, commonly known as jhola-chhaap doctors. These ad-hoc rural healthcare providers had become the first line of treatment.

A quack is typically a male who has spent substantial time assisting qualified doctors or working in hosptials before starting his own rural clinic; he is essentially a layman with an elementary knowledge of medicine.

Although there is no concrete data on the exact number of quacks in India, a 2018 report published in *Mint* estimated that over 1 million quacks were active in the country at the time.[1] In Bihar, which has over 44,000 villages and a predominantly rural population, more than 400,000 quacks are estimated to be operating. In comparison, West Bengal is estimated to have around 100,000 quacks. The numbers for Bihar are significantly higher than those for other states.[2]

The quacks outnumber qualified doctors in India's heartland, where healthcare is often inadequate.

Bihar consistently struggles with a low doctor to population ratio. According to the data released by the Directorate of State Health Services and the National Health Profile in 2018, Bihar had the lowest ratio of doctors to population in the country, with one government-employed doctor for every 28,391 people, compared to the national average of one for every 11,082 people.[3]

This shortage paved the way for quacks to step in, especially in rural areas with little to no medical infrastructure. Since the lockdown was imposed in 2020, the reliance on quacks only increased significantly.

The trust and respect quacks command within rural communities is surprising. During the peak of the second wave, villagers saw them as their only hope, even though they frequently misdiagnosed COVID as typhoid or fever, leading to delays in appropriate treatment, and, in some cases, resulting in death.

But district hospitals were a complete nightmare for people. Take Arrah's only COVID hospital, for example. Infected patients lay on the floor with no nurses in sight. Six ventilators, purchased with PM CARES funds, remained locked in a room because no one was trained to use them. X-ray and CT scan machines also lay unused in locked rooms.

The situation at Sadar Hospital was so dire that Munna Chaudhary, an attendant, told me, 'We drove all the way from Aurangabad, over 110 km from Arrah, to Sadar, but the situation here is so grim. Patients are returning to their villages because the staff refuses to care for them. I've been monitoring my brother-in-law's oxygen levels myself.'

An official from the district administration was equally frustrated.

'We don't even have enough ward boys to clean the hospital. No one wants to wear a PPE kit for hours on end while working. Workers leave after four days in the COVID ward. There is an acute shortage of staff.'

Even fifty km away from the Sadar Hospital, word had spread that it was nothing short of hell.

To learn more about the villages, we drove to the Sahar block, where, in Pirhap village, I met the sarpanch, Satish Sharma.

'Jo hospital ja raha hai, woh wapis nahin aa raha. Toh logon nc ghar par hi treatment karna shuru kar diya,' he told me. (Whoever is going to the hospital isn't returning alive, so people have started getting treatment at home.)

In the last forty-five days, thirty people had died of COVID in his village.

'There is no point rushing to towns now,' Sharma said.

As we walked through the village lanes, we saw returned migrants and farmers gathering for their evening chats. COVID-was the main topic of discussion. We knocked on many doors to check on villagers. Along the way, we encountered a quack named Sipahi. He introduced himself as a doctor practising in the village.

We followed him into the house of a sixty-five–year–old woman suffering from gastric issues, despite consistently taking the medicines Sipahi had prescribed on his last visit.

'I always carry medicines like paracetamol, Azithral, Chloramphenicol and Vitamin C tablets with me, so that I can treat people anywhere,' Sipahi told us. He gave the woman some new pills since the previous ones hadn't worked, and instructed her son to ensure she took them on time.

Sipahi wasn't the only quack in Pirhap. Another one, Sourab Kumar Sharma, also worked there. Both had built a dedicated and loyal patient base over the years.

Sourab Kumar Sharma had gained experience by working at Arrah's Sadar Hospital, observing doctors and nurses for a long time, before starting his own practice. 'I was an ICU in-charge at Arrah's Sadar Hospital for two years,' he said.

Back in my village—Rasulpur in the Mahendragarh district of Haryana—too, people were falling sick.

My mother shared various conspiracy theories that she had heard while working in the fields.

'Beta, bukhar ho rakhya hai sabke. Koi kahe hai ki China ne ye bukhar apne desh mein chhod diya,' she told me over the phone. (Everyone has a fever. Some say that China has spread this fever in our country.)

Thirty kilometres from my village in Haryana is Manethi, where my bua (paternal aunt) lives. She also spoke of a mysterious fever that had gripped her village.

'Typhoid ho gaya hai logon ko.' (People have contracted typhoid.)

With no testing facilities available in the villages, people called it different names—a mysterious fever, typhoid—or even thought it to be just a common cold.

Far away from home, I was anxious for my folks in Haryana. In my dreams, I saw only dead bodies, SOS messages and hospitals. My phone gallery now had over a 1,000 photos of cremation grounds, dead bodies strewn in hospitals and grieving families.

Back in Pirhap, upon seeing us, the villagers covered their faces with gamchhas. They had heard that surgical masks carried germs and could cause disease, so they preferred gamchhas.

'Modi-ji bhi gamchha pahante hain. Unko virus kuch nahi karega toh humko kya karega.' (Even Modi-ji wears a gamchha. If the virus doesn't affect him, it won't affect us either.)

Arrah, a rural district with twelve blocks and a population of 27 lakh, had fifty-four active cases on 5 April 2021. By 9 May, the number had risen to 830. Yet, the district was testing only about 2,000 samples a day on an average. A large section of the rural population was suffering from COVID-like symptoms, yet only a limited number of test samples were collected. The reported active cases reflected only those within the sample group, while countless others were left unaccounted for.

District Magistrate Roshan Kushwaha insisted that patients coming to Sadar Hospital were not being turned away.

'Even if we don't have a bed, we will provide oxygen. We have patients coming from Patna and Bihta as well. We have also roped in six private hospitals. But the numbers have been overwhelming for the past fifteen days.'

When asked about the rural population left to fend for themselves, he replied, 'For the rural belt, we have primary health centres and community health centres. We have prepared kits with treatment protocol medicines. We are testing people at the village level and distributing the kits.'

As Sajid and I travelled to other villages, we consistently observed quacks treating the patients with COVID-like symptoms.

We met a general physician in Khaira market, who introduced himself as Dr Mukesh Kumar. Khaira is a town located approximately thirty km away from the Arrah district headquarters.

'I treat 90 per cent of them. They recover with the help of the COVID-19 medicine kit. But the remaining 10 per cent have breathing problems. I refer them to Sadar hospital.'

Dr Mukesh Kumar ran a makeshift clinic in a shuttered shop with just a bench for patients to sit on. Located in a lane at the back of the market, his clinic, despite its dubious appearance, had become a lifeline during the second wave.

We also tracked down a quack named Mangal Singh, who was operating from the same market as Dr Mukesh Kumar.

'I wanted to become a doctor, either by studying or practicing medicine,' Singh told us. Mangal Singh couldn't get into a medical college and ended up with a bachelor's degree in Zoology. He now introduced himself as Dr Mangal Singh, and made a decent living as a quack.

When we spoke to the district magistrate, he mentioned plans to circulate two-minute video clips by renowned doctors in the district on how to handle mild COVID-19 cases. This initiative aimed to educate not only government-affiliated rural healthcare workers but also the quacks.

The next day (9 May), Sajid and I reached the village Kuber Chakdandhiya, fifteen km from Arrah. There, we met Ram Pravesh Yadav, who was showing symptoms. When he first mentioned feeling sick, his son Anil had taken him to the nearest primary health centre in Koelwar, only to return home disappointed. He then tried the local clinics, but no doctor was willing to see his father.

'Doctor logan dekhat naikhe. Sab haath khade kar diye hain.' (The doctors refused to examine my father. They have washed their hands of the case.)

After being turned away by several doctors in town, a pharmacist came to his rescue.

He gave Anil Vitamin C, Zinc, Azithromycin and paracetamol—the common drugs and supplements prescribed for COVID symptoms.

When I met Anil on 9 May, his father was lying on a cot, still coughing. But Anil was hopeful that he would recover soon.

'I am thankful to the chemist,' he said.

'This is the case in every home in the village. No one has access to doctors in towns. They simply refuse to see the patient if we mention fever and cough.'

Kuber Chakdandhiya was a small village, with a population of 1,300. It had recorded four deaths since 1 April 2021. While in the neighbouring village of Kulharia, with a population of 12,000, twenty-five people had died in the same time period.[4]

There, every person in the village head's joint family of fifteen showed symptoms.

When they insisted that I have tea with them, I had to remind them that they might have COVID and they should isolate themselves.

'Mukhiya ji ka mizaaj theek nahin hai,' one of the village elders sitting outside Mukhiya Surender Yadav's home said.

In rural Bihar, COVID-19 became a disease with no name. Most villagers simply described their condition as 'mizaaj theek nahin hai' (not feeling well).

'What more can we do?' wondered Surender Yadav. 'We are not an isolated case. Every household has patients. Most of them recover, but a few succumb to the illness too. There is no testing facility in the village. So we don't know for sure if it's COVID or not. What's worrying is that the town's doctors have shut their clinics. …

Gaon dehat asahaay ho jata agar ye jhola-chhaap doctor nahin aate.' (The villagers would have been rendered helpless if these quacks hadn't come to our aid.)

It was his family 'doctor' who came to his assistance when Arrah's Sadar and other local private hospitals in the district—the former overburdened and the latter shut down—didn't.

15

The COVID Orphans

It was time to part ways with Sajid as he had other stories to chase. And Babloo, unfamiliar with the roads in Bihar, also decided to leave.

I travelled to Begusarai with my third driver, Binod, a local from Patna.

I had arranged to follow a testing team in one of Begusarai's blocks. The Collector, Arvind Kumar Verma, had connected me with an SDM to facilitate this.

At this time, bodies of abandoned COVID victims were found floating in the Ganga in Ghazipur, Uttar Pradesh and Buxar, Bihar. My editor asked me to return to Buxar, but I was already in Begusarai. So, Sajid was sent to Buxar, while I tried to find out who was abandoning these bodies.

I dropped the testing team story and travelled to Mokama, a neighbouring town and municipal council in Patna district, to meet a Manjhi family who had to bury a woman in the Ganga because they couldn't afford the last rites.

'She complained of chest pain and breathlessness, and died,' the family told me. This was a small hamlet inhabited by the Manjhi community, situated in a secluded corner of the village, segregated from other communities. The area lacked basic amenities such as drainage and sanitation, and most of the houses were kutcha huts.

The family waited until late evening to bury her in the Ganga. They didn't want to be seen dropping the body into the river, so they put her in a sack and filled it with sand to ensure it wouldn't float up. I drove to the spot on the riverbank where the family had buried her. There were signs of other bodies having been submerged in the river.

The Manjhi family explained that buying wood and other essentials for the last rites would have cost at least 4,000–5,000 rupees. Due to the lockdown, the family was out of work. Borrowing such a large sum would only push them further into debt. When I asked if they would have done the same in ordinary times, they quickly said no.

Before I could find more families in similar situations—unable to afford testing, treatment or last rites—Bihar's then State Water Resources Minister, Sanjay Kumar Jha, posted an alarming tweet, blaming Uttar Pradesh for the dead bodies found floating on the Ganga in Bihar.

He wrote, 'CM Nitish Kumar is pained by both the tragedy and the harm done to River Ganga. He has always been particular about the purity and uninterrupted flow of the river and has asked the administration to intensify patrolling to ensure this is not repeated.'[1]

After reading the tweet, I was certain that publishing the families' names and social backgrounds could lead to the police booking them under the Disaster Management Act or Epidemic Act. I had to drop this story as it could land the poor Manjhis in trouble.

By evening, I returned to Begusarai and resumed work on the testing team story.

I received an image on WhatsApp—a clipping from a local Hindi daily. The headline said a girl had to bury her parents in a field because no one from the village came forward to help her. At first glance, the girl looked like a healthcare worker, dressed in a PPE kit, with her face covered, the image was heartwrenching.

I pitched the idea to my editor, and after receiving approval, I immediately left for Araria district—the home of the girl in the news clipping.

The BDO of Raniganj block connected me to the village head, who then shared several details about the village.

I had expected Binod to be familiar with every corner of Bihar, but it turned out that this was his first time travelling in Seemanchal, he had no knowledge of any of the routes.

For most ground reporters, drivers not only take them from one place to another but also serve as guides and point persons. For digital journalists, they often double as cameramen. For a female reporter travelling alone, a driver is not just the first point of contact in unfamiliar towns and villages, but also a crucial safety net.

Since Binod didn't know the routes, I relied on Google Maps to navigate. It was 11 in the morning when I left, and I was tired. This was my thirty-fourth day on the road.

We were about a dozen kilometres away from the Bishanpur panchayat where the COVID orphans lived. The village head was constantly guiding me over the phone.

The route to Bishanpur passed through a small cluster of villages.

Suddenly, Binod slowed down in a busy lane. A few shops were closed, and people were sitting outside them.

A young man banged on our car's door. Judging by his face, he probably wasn't even twenty.

I thought he might know Binod. The man spoke to him in a mix of Maithili and Bhojpuri; I understood parts of the conversation. He was asking Binod to follow him.

Binod didn't know the man. He was asking us to follow him because he needed help.

Binod's window was rolled down. The young man had stuck his hand in and wasn't letting him roll it up.

He said there had been an accident and as media persons we should go to the site.

I told him to let us pass.

Within a minute, another man appeared, just as young. I got nervous as the conversation heated up and the men blocked our way.

Without clearly explaining why they had stopped the vehicle, they kept murmuring to the people standing around. When I intervened, they dismissed me, saying they were talking to my driver, not me. Then they threatened to drag him out. When I sensed that they were trying to instigate a mob against us, I started making frantic calls.

The Collector of Araria was on leave and I hadn't informed the SP that I was coming. I called other officials in the surrounding districts

A mob had gathered around the car by now. Soon, the men left the driver alone and came after me.

Those were the scariest ten minutes of my life. I had never felt so vulnerable. Tears welled up in my eyes, but putting on a brave face, I said to one of the men that I was travelling alone and they were making me feel unsafe.

The men then started accusing Binod of hitting a woman, claiming that she had died.

I asked Binod to somehow get us out of this situation. My fear was that it could escalate to sexual violence.

I was frozen with fear.

One of the district magistrates finally managed to reach the SP, Hridyakant.

Hridyakant asked personnel from the nearest police station to reach the spot in order to escort me safely out of that village.

The two aggressors overheard our conversation, and when I asked them to come to the nearest police station, they changed the subject, and started blabbering incoherently.

We drove for twenty minutes without slowing down at speed breakers. I kept looking back to check if the men were following us. The police met us on a small bridge and we trailed behind their jeep. I was confused when their car stopped after a short distance. Apparently, they were out of fuel. 'Madam, itna hi petrol tha, baaki ab jeb se bharna padega,' one of the policemen said. (Madam, we had only so much petrol, now we'll have to buy more out of our own pocket.)

They instantly reminded me of the policemen from Sonia Faleiro's book *The Good Girls: An Ordinary Killing*, where she described officers from UP who had no money to put fuel in their vehicles.

Fortunately, the mukhiya of Bishanpur had arrived by then, so I thanked the policemen and left with the mukhiya.

In Bishanpur, the orphaned children waited for me, along with about fifty other people.

My first thought was, where were these people when the children needed them? Is COVID suddenly not a concern?

But at least they were wearing cloth masks.

The man who had brought us to the village actually turned out to be the village head's relative.

I took the children into their house and sat on the verandah floor. It took some time for them to open up, but once they did, I was in tears.

'We sold two of our goats for 11,000 rupees and our cow for 10,000 to pay for my parents' treatment,' said nineteen-year-old Soni Kumari, the oldest of the three siblings.

'But even after spending 2,50,000 rupees, most of which we had borrowed, we couldn't save them.'

Soni and her two siblings, fifteen-year-old Nitish Kumar and twelve-year-old Chandni, had lost their mother soon after their father.

'After our father died, no one would lend us any more money. He was the sole earning member of the family, and with him gone, people were apprehensive about whether we would be able to repay the loan. We were forced to discontinue our mother's treatment at the hospital in Raniganj, and she too passed away on 7 May,' Soni added.

Her brother sat on a cot, playing on their father's phone. Their father had died just four days ago. The siblings had brought their mother home from the hospital when they realised they couldn't afford her treatment. When her condition became critical, they tried to rush her back, but she died on the way.

With the fear of COVID spreading through the village like wildfire, Soni and her siblings were left to cope with their loss alone. The villagers kept a safe distance from the family.

Soni, Nitish and Chandni had to arrange a hurried burial.

They showed me their mother's favourite spots in the house—where she sat, where she ate. Their father's bike remained parked outside, and the small medicine shop he ran was locked up. The house was mostly plastered with mud. Only some parts were made of concrete, others were kutcha.

I then asked Soni, 'Where are the fields?'

Soni and Chandni escorted me along a trail to the fields, about 500 metres from their house.

As we walked, Chandni reminisced, 'Ab ghar soona lagta hai. Itne saal saath guzare toh ab samajh nahin aa raha kuch.' (We spent our entire lives with our parents. The house feels empty without them; we don't know anything anymore).

The girls referred to the graves as 'mummy' and 'papa'. They removed their slippers and touched the ground with affection and reverence.

'The one near the tree is mummy's, and the other is our father's.' Soni gestured towards the graves. When we returned from the fields, Chandni said, 'Papa dead kiya toh kisi ne khana tak nahin khilaya humko.' (After our father died, no one even offered us any food.)

Bishanpur village panchayat, located about 350 km from Patna, comprises fourteen wards. Soni's parents—forty-six-year-old Birendra Mehta and thirty-eight-year-old Priyanka Devi—were residents of Ward No. 7, along with 373 other families.

At the beginning of May 2021, the ward had reported seven COVID cases, including Birendra and his wife. The other five patients remained in home quarantine.

Birendra and Priyanka had big dreams for their children. Birendra Mehta, though a quack, had managed to make some money. Like thousands of other quacks, he had learnt medicine through practice. The family belonged to the Koeri caste, classified as a 'Backward Caste' in Bihar.

The couple, who had studied only up to class eight, wanted their children to get an education and become officers. To inspire them, they had named their son after the state's chief minister, Nitish Kumar, who belonged to the same caste as them. Soni and Chandni asked me to tell Nitish Kumar this if I ever met him.

Chandni pointed to the refrigerator their father had bought in 2017. 'He used to say that we would build a big pucca house soon.'

The siblings told me that the day their mother died en route to the hospital, the panchayat mukhiya, Saroj Kumar Mehta, said, 'It's not safe to bring a COVID body home.'

The mukhiya, himself COVID positive, used to go on evening walks and chat freely with people, quarantining himself only during the day.

When I visited his home, he insisted that I have tea with him. The rules for COVID patients in villages were based on convenience. In some places, a COVID positive person would be boycotted, while in others, they could walk around freely.

So, when Soni and her siblings were told that they couldn't cremate their parents' bodies, they took them to the nearby field and buried them there, four days apart.

'The villagers said if we cremate the bodies, the whole area will be infected. So it is better to bury them. My cousins dug the graves.

No one came to pay their last respects, and I buried my mother beside my father,' Soni said.

Nitish tried to help his sisters. He carried his father's phone, answering calls from NGOs and social activists offering help.

The siblings claimed to have started receiving monetary assistance from people after their posts went viral on social media.

'We have received around 2,000 messages from the bank, informing us of the money people have sent. But we are currently busy with the shradh preparations, we'll visit the bank afterwards,' said Soni.

I wanted to find out how her parents, who never went to the city during the pandemic, contracted the virus in the first place.

As I delved into this, I discovered that Bihar, like the rest of the country, was still holding public weddings and funerals. Soni's parents had attended Birendra's father in law's funeral on 16 April in Purnea district.

In other villages, the virus had spread through migrants who had returned for Holi at the end of March as well as after the lockdown was announced again in April.

'Most of us contracted COVID from migrant workers who returned to the villages from different states during Holi or after lockdowns were imposed there. Many here attended funerals of people who had died of some mysterious illness in adjoining areas,' the village head Saroj Mehta told me.

A week after attending that funeral, Soni's father developed a fever and cough.

On 27 April, his condition worsened, and he tested positive on 1 May. Priyanka also tested positive, but the three children, whose samples were taken on 5 May, tested negative.

'We took my father to Raniganj hospital. He was then referred to Forbesganj, and Forbesganj referred him to Purnea Sadar. In two days, the hospitals passed him around so much that he died,' said Soni.

'Babu, hum nahin bachbo, hum mar jaibo.' (I won't survive, I will die.) Chandni recalled her mother's last words.

'We received the COVID-19 death certificate for my mother, so the district administration has given us a cheque for 4 lakh rupees as compensation,' said Soni, referring to the Bihar government's compensation scheme for families of COVID victims.

'But at the time of my father's death, we were not in the right frame of mind. We left the hospital without getting the certificate. The BDO, though, has promised that we will be given help.' However, Chandni said, 'Kitna bhi paisa milega, ma-baap to nahin milega na.' (No matter how much money we get, we are not going to get our parents back.)

A week before my visit to Araria, the Union Ministry of Women and Child Development (WCD) had instructed the health ministry to ensure that hospitals took declarations from parents being admitted about the guardianship of their children in the event of their death. Unfortunately, this directive came too late to help Birendra Mehta and Priyanka's family.

I contacted Atul Prasad, the Additional Chief Secretary of Bihar WCD, to learn more about the state government's approach to COVID orphans.

'The Bihar government has a scheme called Parvarish Yojana, under which such children will be cared for in childcare homes,' he said, noting that the primary concern in such cases was to ensure the children did not fall prey to trafficking.

Meanwhile, Soni and her siblings were busy arranging their parents' shradh on 16 May, expecting close relatives to attend it. Struggling to cope with the weight of their loss, the three had not considered their future. Money was the last thing on their minds when I met them.[2]

Later, as life began to stabilise, they started sending me messages every once in a while, video-calling me from their father's phone and inviting me to visit them.

'Didi, when will you come to see us?' they would ask. Each time, I would explain that I was writing about children like them, but in another part of the country.

On the policy front, Bihar's Chief Minister Nitish Kumar launched financial aid of Rs 1,500 per month for children who lost either parent to COVID under the 'Bal Sahayata Yojana'.

Additionally, orphans without guardians would be taken to children's homes, and girls would be enrolled in the Kasturba Gandhi residential schools.

This initiative was in addition to the state government's provision of 4 lakh rupees as ex-gratia to the next of kin of each person who died of COVID.[3]

As more stories of COVID orphans surfaced across the country, Prime Minister Narendra Modi responded by announcing the PM CARES for Children scheme on 29 May 2021. This scheme aimed to support children who had lost their biological parents, legal guardians or adoptive parents to the pandemic between 11 March 2020 and 28 February 2022.

It mandated financial assistance through a monthly stipend until the children turned eighteen, and a lump sum of 10 lakh rupees, accessible when they turned twenty-three. Additionally, it offered support for accommodation, health insurance and education.

According to the Bal Swaraj portal, established in May 2021 by the National Commission for Protection of Child Rights (NCPCR), 153,827 children had been either orphaned or left with a single parent, or abandoned during the pandemic as of 15 February 2022.[4] This data was released by the government in response to a study published by the UK-based medical journal, *The Lancet Child & Adolescent Health*, which reported that over 5.2 million children across twenty-one countries lost one or both parents to COVID.[5]

According to this study, the age group most affected ranged from ten to seventeen years. The highest rates of orphaned children were reported in Peru, South Africa, Mexico and India. India alone was estimated to have approximately 1.9 million COVID orphans, accounting for 36.54 per cent of the global sum.

However, in March 2022, the Women and Child Development Minister, Smriti Irani disputed this estimate, stating that the data released by the Indian government was twelve times lower than *The Lancet*'s figures. The press release was titled 'Lancet Article Sophisticated Trickery Intended to Create Panic Among Citizens, Divorced from Truth and Ground Reality.[6]'

The Lancet's study claimed that the pandemic had orphaned as many children in two years as HIV/AIDS had done in ten.

In July 2024, the Women and Child Development Ministry released national data on the PM CARES for Children scheme. A total of 9,331 applications were received from 613 districts across thirty-three states and union territories (UTs).[7] Of these, only 4,532 applications from 558 districts in thirty-two states and UTs were approved, while 4,781 applications were rejected and 18 were pending approval. This means that 51 per cent of the applications were rejected.

States such as Rajasthan, Maharashtra and Uttar Pradesh received the highest number of applications: 1,553, 1,511 and 1,007, respectively.

Bihar received approval for only ninety orphaned children under the PM CARES for Children scheme. Among these, twenty-nine children had lost both parents. According to the data accessed from the Bihar government, ninety-four orphaned children were identified by the state and provided with a monthly allowance of 1,500 rupees until they turned eighteen. Thirty of these children reached eighteen years of age by October 2024.

The state spent ₹9.90 lakh on the scheme in 2022–23, ₹12.60 lakh in 2023–24 and ₹5.17 lakh in 2024–25, totalling ₹27.67 lakh on monthly allowances for COVID orphans.

In 2023, Soni got married at the age of twenty-one. She married into a neighbouring village within the same panchayat. She's now a mother. The sudden loss of her parents and the responsibilities that fell on her shoulders in the aftermath forced her to drop out of school after class ten.

'My husband has now enrolled me in class eleven,' Soni told me, cradling her newborn.

Nitish relocated to Purnea town in 2023 to continue his education in a private school. As for Chandni's education, although she enrolled in class eleven at the government school in the panchayat, she has temporarily moved to live with her mausi (maternal aunt) in Purnea district.

Nitish plans to study medicine, but not by getting an MBBS degree. Instead, he intends to learn pathology by working with a doctor and, with years of practice, become a pathologist.

'Jaanch karna hai,' he told me, explaining that he has arranged to work with a local doctor in Line Bazaar, Purnea. If Nitish's plan succeeds, he will join the ranks of thousands of pathologists working in small towns across Bihar without a diploma or a degree, in various laboratories, hospitals and private clinics.

As far as the compensation is concerned, Nitish and Chandni both received 10 lakh rupees under the PM CARES for Children Scheme. Soni, being over eighteen years of age at the time, was not eligible. They also received 4 lakh rupees ex gratia from the Bihar government for their mother's death. But their father's death certificate was never released by the hospital, so they couldn't qualify for the additional 4 lakh rupees' ex gratia.

Additionally, they received 1,500 rupees per month from the Bihar government. Nitish's allowance has been stopped now that he is eighteen, but Chandni still receives it.

Nitish told me that their bank account details were posted on social media by social workers, journalists and local activists in the aftermath of his parents' death. People contributed generously, raising a substantial sum of nine to ten lakh rupees. The siblings used this money to repay the debt they had run up for their parents' treatment and Soni's dowry and wedding expenses (which amounted to around four to five lakhs), and to fund Nitish's education in Purnea.

Returning to the incident involving the two young men: I had just met the children and was on my way to Purnea district. I couldn't sleep that night as images of being chased by those men haunted me.

For the next three days, I disconnected from the news cycle. The experience had left me badly shaken. For a week or so, I lived in mortal fear of men. I had managed to take a photograph of them, in case I needed to report the incident to the police.

After narrating the incident to my editor, Shekhar Gupta, I told him that I wanted to return to Delhi immediately. He said I could return anytime. And in case I decided to stay on, he suggested I always take a local reporter or stringer along to unfamiliar places.

After this experience, I started dropping messages to the SPs or collectors, informing them of my assignments whenever I arrived in their districts. This way, I could reach out in case of any emergencies.

At the end of our conversation, Shekhar encouraged me to take a short break before continuing with my assignments. Which I did. But I also decided to file a complaint. Araria SP Hridyakant asked me to share the photos I had taken to help track down the men.

A few days later, he informed me that both the men had been apprehended. They apologised, and since they had no prior criminal record, I chose not to pursue the case further.

But I kept wondering afterwards why they had targeted me. I began to connect the dots between their actions and the broader issues affecting the youth in Seemanchal Bihar (Eastern Bihar), the districts of Purnea, Katihar, Araria and Kishanganj. According to the 2011 census, around one crore people lived in the region at the time. Out of which, around 25 lakh fell within the age group of fifteen to twenty-four.

In March 2022, I travelled to this region to report on the rampant drug abuse among the youth. People spoke about the 'red-eyed, thin, lost young men' in their area.[8]

One could spot them in mango orchards, closed school buildings, abandoned historical sites, dark city lanes and even cremation grounds. They picked fights, snatched mobile phones or gold chains and some even stole hand pumps, to make a quick buck and buy drugs.

What triggered this Punjab-like situation in rural eastern Bihar? According to families, officials and the drug addicts themselves, Nitish Kumar's 2016 liquor ban played a significant role. Heroin, ganja, charas and intravenous drugs became easy alternatives. An UDAYA study found that drug consumption was higher among rural boys (21 per cent of the total respondents) in Bihar as compared to the youth in urban areas (17 per cent).[9]

Police officials in Seemanchal's districts pointed out that petty crimes had become more frequent, as had the recovery of drugs, stolen phones and cough syrup bottles in recent years. The story of drug abuse in Bihar was published in my series titled 'Generation Nowhere'. The term was first used by scholar Craig Jeffrey to describe how educated, unemployed youth in India spent their days.[10]

With our system plagued by paper leaks in competitive government job exams, shrinking salaries, army jobs on hold for years before the Agniveer scheme, cheap 2GB data and with the clamping down on campus politics across Indian universities, young minds have been increasingly turning to cyber crimes, drug abuse and other misdemeanours. Millions of youngsters have lost hope, and this crisis is reshaping India and its politics. 'Generation Nowhere' was an attempt to read young India's mind.

Each year, the economically backward Seemanchal sends its sons to Delhi, Mumbai and other big cities for better education and jobs.

Some leave as migrant workers and some as government job seekers. The number is in lakhs. When the nationwide lockdown was announced in 2020, many young migrant workers, government job aspirants and college students returned home with no jobs in hand. With that, entered boredom, and different types of addictions. The proximity to borders with Nepal and Bengal fuelled Bihar's drug culture.

When I travelled by road through Seemanchal, I noticed posters and graffiti in many places, which issued warnings: 'Madyapaan varjit hai' (consuming liquor is prohibited). The state's focus had not yet shifted to the growing abuse of drugs among the youth. All awareness campaigns, marathons and community police initiatives of the state were still predominantly focused on alcohol.

This likely explained why most of the de-addiction centres in the state's district hospitals were dysfunctional. I visited four de-addiction centres in Seemanchal, only to find them closed. These centres were established in 2016 when the state had banned liquor.

16

If There Is a Hell, It Is Here

After a four-hour drive from Purnea, we reached Darbhanga late in the evening on 15 May.

During the first wave, our coverage had taken us directly from Sitamarhi to Katihar, bypassing many significant districts. This time, I wanted to report from the very heart of the Mithilanchal region—Darbhanga.

The government buildings were adorned with beautiful Madhubani art. We stayed at the circuit house. Since it was almost fully occupied, I was given a rather old room, situated in the farthest corner of the old building. The room had a tall ceiling, a fan with a long rod and huge, airy doors. I found the oldness quite charming.

Darbhanga is connected to the state capital, Patna, via NH22 and NH27. A three-hour drive brings you to this historically and culturally rich town, once the seat of Darbhanga Raj, ruled by the Khandwalas, a prominent Maithil Brahmin dynasty. They ruled over 10,360 square kilometres of land between India and Nepal and were considered one of the largest and richest Zamindaris in British India.

Today, Darbhanga is a district. With a population of about 40 lakhs, it comprises three sub-divisions and eighteen blocks, and hosts ten assembly seats and one Lok Sabha seat.

On the morning of 16 May, I arranged a meeting with the then district magistrate, Thiyagarajan S.M. to get administrative insights. The area surrounding the Collectorate lacked the usual bustle and was rather quiet. I headed straight to his chamber.

The district magistrate, a lean man with a serious demeanour, sat across from me. On my way to the collectorate, I had scrolled through a few tweets from Delhi-based senior journalist Narendra Nath Mishra, who hailed from the region. He had been writing about the shortage of basic medicines like paracetamol in his home district. I asked about it and Thiyagarajan got upset. The interview barely lasted five minutes. Before I turned to leave, he asked me to meet the deputy development commissioner, Tanay Sultania if I had more questions. With Sultania, my conversation was very cordial; he provided valuable data and insights. I expressed interest in following a doctor around for a day in the COVID ward, and he promised to find one for my next story. The next morning, thanks to Sultania, I received several contact details for doctors from nodal officers and Collector Thiyagarajan seemed okay with it.

I called every doctor on that list. Most declined, one consented to a phone interview, but the goal of the story wasn't just to gather quotes but to capture their vulnerabilities, dilemmas and despair as they spent their days in close proximity to the virus, always at the risk of getting infected, the first to witness large-scale casualty and take the blame.

I thanked her and continued to look for more doctors. I had no luck.

Meanwhile, a photograph of Darbhanga Medical College & Hospital (DMCH) was circulating on social media, showing the building in a deplorable condition. I asked Binod to drive me there. Upon arrival, I discovered that the photograph was indeed of the old buildings of DMCH, but taken a while ago.

Now, DMCH was operating out of three functional units spread across three different buildings, out of which two had been transformed into isolation wards for patients who needed oxygen support and standard treatment, while the third was dedicated to patients who required ventilator support.

It was the fourth building, the Old Surgery Wing, whose photograph had gone viral. Contrary to the claims on Twitter, this ward was not used for treating COVID patients but served as a transition area. If a patient arrived at DMCH and no beds were available, they would be kept in the Old Surgery Wing for a few days before being transferred to the isolation ward. The waiting period could range from one to five days.

The Old Surgery Wing, once the site of major surgeries, had fallen into severe disrepair. Paint had peeled off its walls, the roof seemed to be on the verge of collapse, its wards had been devastated by floods and long wild grass crept up the building's exterior, giving it an eerie, abandoned look.

When I stood in the middle of this wing, the last few COVID-positive patients were being transferred to another building designated as a COVID facility. I followed the patients and their attendants to the new location, only to discover that the conditions there were even worse than the viral image that had sparked outrage on social media. In fact, this was the worst I had ever seen.

In the new facility, as the clock struck 5 p.m., a loud moan echoed through Ward No. 3—one of the isolation wings for COVID patients—its pitch high enough to drown out the grunts of pigs roaming outside, and to put other patients and their families on edge.

Manoj Kumar Yadav, helplessly rubbed his father's back to give him some relief. But his efforts were of little help to the old man gasping for breath—the patient's oxygen cylinder wasn't working.

A team of four doctors, checking on the patients, bypassed Ward No. 3.

Five painful minutes passed before the doctors returned accompanied by four nurses. One of the doctors fixed the oxygen supply, another checked his pulse, the third one tried to revive the old man and a nurse left to fetch an injection for him.

The condition of the hospital was bound to make one pity the desperation of those who were forced to admit their people here.

As if the pigs roaming just outside the hospital wasn't bad enough, one found dogs sleeping inside the corridors, lizards raced across the walls and the stench of cow dung pervaded the decrepit old building.

The filthy toilets, with no separate facilities for women, forced women to relieve themselves in the dim corners of the corridors. There was little light in the wing, and the attendants accompanying patients often relied on the torchlight from their phones. There were no ceiling fans either, so they brought table fans.

The nurses' chamber did not have proper ventilation.

This was a hospital serving at least five districts in north Bihar—Darbhanga, Samastipur, Madhubani, Begusarai and Supaul—with a combined population of 2.5 crores.

Fortunately, there was no shortage of oxygen here because DMCH had its own oxygen plant which produced about 1,000 cylinders every day. But the hospital had run out of medicines.

'I have had to source antibiotics for my father from outside for the past week,' said Ram Kumar, whose seventy-year-old father, Kailash, was getting treated there for the last twelve days.

'He has undergone COVID tests thrice and the reports have always been negative, but he still needs oxygen support,' Ram Kumar added.

Though he said that the nurses were cooperative, when I visited the hospital for two consecutive days, most patients were being attended to by accompanying family members.

If life here at DMCH was tough, death was without any dignity. Bodies lay unattended for hours, like gloomy shadows, among patients battling severe complications.

I called the Deputy Medical Superintendent of DMCH, Mani Bhushan.

'Doctors and nurses work in three shifts, each shift comprising five doctors and seven nurses. More doctors are being hired based on walk-in interviews,' he said.

According to the district health data shared by the DDC (Deputy Development Commissioner), DMCH had 120 beds with oxygen support in addition to seven ICU beds.

Darbhanga had reported only five fresh COVID cases on 20 April, but by 17 May, the number of active cases in the district had gone up to 1,176.

'The administration has engaged twenty private hospitals to deal with the crisis, and the district currently has 40 beds with ventilator support, of which 35 are in private hospitals,' claimed the DDC.

One of the nurses at DMCH sneaked out to give me a glimpse of the conditions under which they had to work. 'Are we not human?'

A woman, who had accompanied one of the patients in the ward, also tagged along, hoping to find a toilet on the way.

'Ek washroom nahin hai yahaan, hum aath ghante tang hokar baithe rahte hain. Raat ko hum log sadak par isi dress mein jaate hain. Ek pehra deti hai.' (There isn't a single toilet for women here. We work eight hour-shifts like this. In the evening, we go out in twos to relieve ourselves along the roadside. One of us stands guard),' the nurse said.

The toilets, she said, were so filthy that 'even an animal wouldn't enter'. They were indeed so filthy that even stray dogs sat at a distance.

The nurses' chamber—crawling with lizards and insects—was in the same state of neglect as the rest of the isolation wing.

Opposite the isolation ward stood an under construction multi-story trauma centre.

Funded with Rs 150 crore from the central government, this centre could have alleviated much of the suffering during the second wave had it been operational.

However, like many government projects, it faced delays for various reasons. The construction had begun in 2016, and despite numerous letters from the hospital administration to local MPs and MLAs requesting a quick handover, the building remained unfinished. Though 90 per cent complete, there was no water supply, making it useless for COVID patients.

Twenty-five–year–old Manoj Kumar from Madhubani district waited on the ground floor of the old surgery wing for a bed for his mother Sunita in the isolation ward. Sunita had been brought to the hospital's emergency ward a day before.

The oldest nurse at DMCH, who had been working at the hospital since 1983 and was due to retire next year, said that Kumar's family was lucky.

'They had to only wait for one day. Many patients have had to wait for four days. We have twenty beds and most of them were occupied in the last fortnight.'

For years, the old surgery wing had become a symbolic image for the media, representing everything that was wrong with the state's healthcare infrastructure. To avoid further embarrassment and scrutiny, the administration decided to shift to a safer location—the isolation ward.

'We used it (the old surgery ward) as a transition building when we did not have enough beds in Zila school (which had been turned into a COVID treatment facility) or DMCH. The average number of patients waiting there at any given time would be about six to seven. Though old, this ward had all the facilities,' insisted DDC Tanay Sultania.

He did not, however, comment on the condition of the isolation ward or the nurses' room.

Necessity can make many immune to difficult conditions. A few critical non-COVID surgeries were still being conducted in the old surgery ward. An elderly couple's young son was recuperating here after undergoing a non-COVID surgery, and the couple occupied the space outside the toilet, cooking, eating and sleeping there, oblivious to the filth and stench surrounding them.

'Agar Darbhanga mein kahin narak hai toh woh DMCH hi hai,' a family member of a patient who endured four days in the isolation ward said. (If there is hell in Darbhanga, it is at DMCH.)

The attendants' plight continued even after they had lost their loved ones. During my visit to DMCH on 18 May, at around 4 p.m., Ganesh Paswan, sixty-five, passed away in the new COVID facility. The patient next to him had died in the morning. There was no one to help Paswan's son, Sudhir, as he ran about trying to figure out how he could take his father's body for the last rites.

Paswan had tested positive for COVID two days ago.

'Body de diya jata … jo side mein zinda hai usko bhi kharab lagta hai agar bagal mein murda padaa rahe,' said a dejected Sudhir. (If only they gave me his body … Those on the other beds will feel worse with a dead body lying in their midst.)

I returned from the hospital and shared the visuals with my editors in Delhi.

The report titled 'If there's hell … it's here: A day with patients in DMCH, north Bihar's mainstay hospital' was published on 20 May 2021.[1]

Within an hour, the report went viral. Citizens from across the country tagged the chief minister, the health minister of Bihar, and the district magistrate, demanding accountability.

By afternoon, I received a message from the DMCH administration. Written in Hindi and signed by the DMCH superintendent, the statement condemned my report and denied the conditions described. It also threatened to file a complaint against me with the Press Council of India.

Here is the translated version of the statement:

'Correspondent Jyoti Yadav has given absolutely baseless, misleading and false information regarding the COVID ward at DMCH.

It must be noted that correspondent Jyoti Yadav wanted to visit the Corona ward and Corona isolation ward of DMCH. The doctors present there didn't give her permission under the COVID-19 protocols in place. Following this, she misbehaved with officials and doctors there and gave false and misleading information regarding DMCH. DMCH denies and condemns it. DMCH will also file a complaint against correspondent Jyoti Yadav with the Press Council of India.
Superintendent,
DMCH, Darbhanga.'

The next day, *ThePrint* published my response to the absurd rebuttal which falsely accused me of misbehaving with the doctors. *ThePrint* affirmed its support for the report, stating that Darbhanga Hospital's allegation of misconduct by the correspondent was untrue. There was no altercation or unpleasant argument.

Throughout the day, I faced threats, internet trolling and intimidation from the administration. However, my editor, Shekhar Gupta, stood firmly by me.

This was my response to the DMCH:

'The DMCH's allegation that I misbehaved with doctors and officials is completely baseless. I only met DDC Tanay Sultania and District Magistrate Thiyagrajan S.M. in person, and spoke to DMCH officials and doctors only on the phone, and those conversations were cordial. The truth must be stated: Nobody tried obstructing me at all. So, there was no altercation or unpleasant argument.'

I concluded by expressing hope that DMCH would indeed take this matter to the honourable Press Council of India (PCI). Perhaps then, the PCI would send a fact-finding team to Darbhanga to verify the conditions firsthand.

A few days after my report, several national media houses covered the same COVID ward, prompting the administration to publicly commit to improving the conditions within a fortnight.

While the Darbhanga Medical College Hospital was a nightmare for people, lacking basic facilities such as toilets, lights, fans and water, there were also 'showcase' hospitals built using crores of rupees, featuring tall buildings on expansive campuses in the rural landscape. Their infrastructure offered a glimmer of hope, but inside the COVID wards of these Bihar hospitals too, neglect and mismanagement prevailed.

Jan Nayak Karpoori Thakur Medical College and Hospital (JNKTMCH) was inaugurated by Bihar's Chief Minister Nitish Kumar in March 2020. This was part of the government's promise to strengthen the state's healthcare system, ensuring that residents wouldn't need to travel elsewhere for treatment. Named after a former Bihar chief minister, it was built at a cost of ₹800 crore in Madhepura district.

During the first wave, JNKTMCH served as a dedicated COVID facility.

Like DMCH, this hospital is a lifeline for seven adjoining districts in the Kosi-Seemanchal region in northeastern Bihar.

On 12 May, just after covering the COVID orphans story, I visited the hospital. At that time, 83 of its 102 oxygen beds were occupied. According to the hospital administration, it had 50 pulse oximeters, 19 ventilators and 19 ICU beds.

But moderate and critical COVID patients—admitted on the third and fourth floors—were neglected by the staff.

Among these neglected patients was one Laxmi Ram, a forty-five-year-old government school teacher. While I stood outside the COVID ward, noting down my observations, one of Laxmi Ram's sons approached me and asked if I was from the media.

When I confirmed this, he requested that I go inside to hear what his old man had to say.

Laxmi Ram wanted me to record his statement.

'Doctor sahab aa jata to turant humko jaan bach pata. Ilaaj nahin ho raha hai. Doctor sahab hamra kam se kam rahat kari,' he said, predicting his death as he struggled to breathe. (If the doctor examines me, I could be saved. I am not receiving any treatment. Some doctor should at least try to save me.)

Surrounded by four family members who rubbed his body trying to improve his oxygen circulation, Laxmi Ram told me he had given up all hope. He tried to remove his oxygen mask in order to speak but could barely finish his sentences.

'Mar rahe hain, koi ilaaj nahin ho paaya.' (I am dying. I haven't been treated.)

His son was distressed. 'We were sure the big hospital would be able to help us, but his condition has worsened since he got here.'

'Doctor sahab aate nahin hai, unko marne ka darr hai. Bahar se hi likh ke dete hain,' he said. (The doctor doesn't come inside; he is scared of dying. He writes prescriptions from outside the ward.)

'We are helpless, even with all the machines and medicines available here. Every day, we see four–five deaths.'

He was right. After spending a day on all the floors designated for COVID-19 patients, I observed that patients were left unattended for hours, despite repeated calls for assistance by their attendants.

I watched as a nurse was called in to help a breathless woman but she didn't show up for at least an hour.

When I questioned the hospital administration, they denied allegations of neglect but acknowledged that many on the staff had contracted the virus and the hospital employees were scared as a result.

After visiting the hospital, I met with District Magistrate Shyam Bihari Meena who told me that he had inspected the hospital on 11 May and had not observed any neglect.

'I personally have the details of every patient admitted there, from their SpO2 levels to their temperature. In fact, I have deployed three state administration officials in three shifts over there. Additionally, I have attached an ADM (Additional District Magistrate) to the hospital,' he claimed. But the attendants told me they were shooed away during the Collector's inspection, and everyone was on their best behaviour. Once the Collector left, they were called upon to look after their patients.

One hospital staff member, speaking on the condition of anonymity, corroborated the patients' accounts.

A young man in his twenties recounted how his father was sent to the mortuary after being declared dead but when he went to claim the body, he found him alive. After a huge commotion, the patient was moved back to the COVID ward.

'Those ten—fifteen minutes were the most difficult moments of my life. How would I have told my mother all this?'

The administration provided a different version of the story.

'The man created a scene. The patient was being shifted to a different ward, but his attendant thought they were sending him to the mortuary,' Collector Meena explained.

The people present at the COVID ward during the incident confirmed that the man had indeed been declared dead.

On the fourth floor, many attendants fed and massaged their patients. A man, desperate to save his mother grabbed my hand and led me to her bed.

'See her condition. I have been calling the nurses for hours now. They don't check the patient at all,' he said, rubbing his mother's back to help her breathe.

I followed him to the nurse's chamber, some distance away from the COVID ward.

He pleaded with a nurse, hands folded, 'Nurse, unko akhiri saans chal raha hai, ek baar chal kar dekh lijiye na.' (Nurse, she is on her last breath, please come and see her once.)

The nurse assured him she would visit and began putting on her PPE kit. I waited outside the COVID ward for an hour, but the nurse never came. At one point, the young man shook his mother to wake her up.

'Itna bada hospital kyon banwaya hai? Ventilator hai, ICU hai, bed hai, oxygen hai. Phir bhi Ma mar rahi hai.' (Why build such a big hospital? It has ventilators, ICUs, beds and oxygen. But my mother is still dying.)

According to the district administration, the hospital was recording four–five COVID deaths every day. His mother was about to become one with those statistics, and no one could do anything to prevent it.

Meanwhile, the medical superintendent was replaced at the peak of the crisis. I tried to meet the new superintendent, Baidyanath Thakur. He explained that the hospital staff was demoralised due to infection among the healthcare workers.

'But nurses not going to the wards … that's not the case,' he claimed.

I shared what I had witnessed firsthand. On the condition of anonymity, a nurse had told me, 'There is a fear of COVID. No one wants to visit the COVID ward and risk dying. We cannot spend the whole day inside the ward.'

The medical superintendent did not comment further on this matter.

17

The Last Leg

In the third week of May, I was still travelling in Mithilanchal with the doctors' story on my mind.

Binod was reluctant to drive me to hospitals, so he called the agency in Patna, making excuses about a wedding he had to attend. When he refused to drive to Madhubani district, I requested him to stay on for just a few more days before his replacement arrived.

Having already faced harassment in Araria, I made it a point to meet District Magistrate Amit Kumar at the Madhubani headquarters first, just to let him know that I'd be in the district and reach out if I needed help. The lockdown was still in effect.

At the Collectorate, Amit was addressing local journalists. When I shared the story I was doing on doctors, he connected me with nodal officers, who in turn connected me with doctors. Finally, I got the story I had been chasing for the last ten days—a day in the life of a doctor in rural Bihar.

That week, the monsoons came knocking on Bihar's door. Mango orchards were heavy with fresh harvest. The fragrance of rain spread throughout the district.

Amidst the rain, ambulances ferried patients and the deceased. I drove to the COVID care hospital to meet thirty-seven-year-old Dr Pankaj Kumar. He had earned his MBBS degree from Bhagalpur, MD from Banaras Hindu University (BHU) and completed his senior residency at Delhi AIIMS. He had been posted at this COVID facility during the first wave.

I sat down with Dr Kumar in a small room that served as a canteen for doctors. They had their meals in separate shifts.

'Sister, ghabrana nahin hai, double vaccinated hain to kuchh toh bachav hai,' Dr Kumar reassured an accompanying nurse. (Sister, don't worry. We have received both the doses, so there's bound to be some protection.)

Just a minute earlier, the nurse, Rachna, had asked Dr Kumar if they would live to see the next year.

'What could I have possibly told her? We are not sure about our own lives now. Each day, we see doctors and nurses succumbing to the virus. There is an uncertainty,' Dr Kumar told me, looking out of the window.

Located eight km from the district headquarters, the nursing college had been converted into a COVID hospital during the first wave. Since then, it had treated all patients from Madhubani district.

Dr Kumar was one among the twenty-five doctors stationed at this hospital. This was his fortieth consecutive day of duty. The hospital could admit 120 patients at a time. On 20 May, eighty-nine patients were admitted.

'The last wave wasn't deadly. This centre reported only one COVID death last year, but there have already been sixty-five deaths in the second surge,' Dr Kumar said.

Doctors and nurses were increasingly getting concerned about their own safety. According to the statistics released by the Indian Medical Association (IMA), 798 doctors died during the second wave. The highest number of deaths was reported in Delhi, where 128 doctors lost their lives. This was followed by Bihar, where 115 doctors died.

When I was reporting this story, ninety-six deaths had already been reported in Bihar, accounting for approximately 29 per cent of the total COVID-related deaths among doctors in the country.

In Madhubani's COVID care facility, the limited infrastructure, the round-the-clock duty of healthcare workers, while also battling the ignorance and hesitation among patients to seek medical aid, added to the frustration of doctors like Kumar.

'We observe critical patients for one day and then if we feel that despite our best efforts, the patient has little chance of survival, we start preparing the family psychologically, telling them things like "Har sambhav prayaas kar rahe hain, oxygen bhi de rahe hain, dawayi bhi jaa rahi hai, we are making all possible efforts, oxygen and medicines are being administered …", and then someone from the family says, "kuchh bhi kijiye, do whatever it takes to save the patient". After that we are left with nothing to say.' To ensure better management and maintain order among distressed families, the district administration had deployed police security and a sub-divisional officer (SDO) at the hospital.

In the middle of our interview, nurses arrived with a PPE kit for me. Until then, I had navigated the COVID wards with just double or triple layers of masks, sometimes a face shield and once even a helmet. This hospital not only allowed me to experience firsthand the challenges faced by doctors in rural areas but was also very supportive in granting access.

We needed to move from one building to another, where COVID patients were admitted. The continuous rains had turned the corridors into muddy, waterlogged paths. Some of the staff members were soaked to the skin. My PPE kit got drenched too. Clicking pictures or jotting down notes in my diary was extremely difficult with gloves on. Somehow, we made it into the COVID ward.

Dr Pankaj, a resident of Samastipur, travelled forty km every day to reach the hospital by 10 a.m.

As the clinical coordinator appointed by the district magistrate, he had additional administrative responsibilities, including liaising with the district magistrate. What he dreaded most were the moments when he had to utter those four heartrenching words, 'he/she is no more'.

As we walked from one room to another, he recounted the story of a forty-year-old teacher whose family had rushed him to the hospital early one morning after he complained of breathlessness.

'His wife was cradling his head in her lap. She thought he was still alive. But I had to tell her that he was already clinically dead,' he told me.

The patient's COVID test results later confirmed he was positive. His wife and ten-year-old son also tested positive.

'What do we say at a moment like this? We have to think of those left behind.'

He added that another constant challenge was the lack of health infrastructure in rural areas.

'Rural areas don't have adequate health infrastructure even in non-COVID times,' he said. With limited resources—including beds, medicines and oxygen supply—Dr Pankaj often found himself struggling to make the best use of what was available.

'This is a level 2 COVID hospital, meaning we have oxygen support but no ventilators or ICU facilities. But most of the patients who come here need level 3 care. We often have to refer them to Darbhanga Medical College & Hospital (DMCH), the larger facility we are officially attached to. But since DMCH is also operating at full capacity, our referred patients often come back to us, and sadly, we are sometimes unable to save them.'

When Dr Pankaj Kumar mentioned DMCH, I shared my experience of reporting from it. He was surprised that the district magistrate had tried to threaten me.

'All of Bihar knows about the condition of DMCH. What is there to misreport?' he asked.

Returning to his own concerns, he mentioned the acute shortage of manpower.

'I often don't even know who the ward boy is, as they keep quitting and new ones keep joining. The nurses at the Rampatti COVID care centre are dedicated, cooperative and well-equipped to handle the situation, because they've been deployed here since the first wave,' he emphasised.

Indeed, the nurses were committed and devoted. But compared to urban setups, what challenges were the doctors and nurses facing? I prodded him for more details.

'The urban belt reacts differently from the rural belt. There is more awareness in cities.'

There is hesitation among rural people about seeking medical help. Hospitals are often visited only when the patient becomes critical. The reasons for this, even in normal times, are varied—financial constraints, lack of education and reliance on unqualified practitioners or quacks. They don't even want to get tested. Then there's the misinformation spread by quacks. They reach out to us at the last stage. Many times, they don't even make it to the COVID ward. They die in the ambulance on the way.' Frustration was evident on Dr Kumar's face.

'Quacks are discouraging people from coming to hospital, which is very concerning,' added another doctor who had been patiently listening to our conversation. He had come for a meal break.

On 20 May, Dr Pankaj spent his day inspecting the COVID ward, trapped in a PPE suit for hours, drenched in sweat and rain.

He adjusted the oxygen supply for one patient, checked another's pulse and comforted distressed families, as I followed him inside the COVID ward.

Tilla Devi, a COVID patient in her sixties, had come to the hospital with an oxygen level of 30. When the doctor approached her bed, she complained to him, 'Saans nahin aa raha, babu.' (I can't breathe, son.)

The term 'babu', common in Bihar and used to convey affection, warmed his heart amidst the bleak medical emergency. Dr Pankaj replied to her in Maithili, telling her to rest and that she would be fine soon.

As he was about to leave the ward, a worried Summy Ahmad, in his twenties, ran up to him and dragged him to his father's bed.

His father was concerned that being prescribed a 'light' meal meant he wasn't recovering. Dr Pankaj reassured them, 'koshish karna hai, theek hona hai.' (You have to try and get well.)

Meanwhile, back home, Dr Pankaj's family spent their days worrying about him.

'If we don't see our family, we will go into depression,' he said, showing pictures of his family on his phone.

Despite the risk of carrying the infection home, he returned every evening during the first and second waves.

The doctor's parents were quarantined in one room of the house, and his two daughters, aged four and seven, were forbidden from hugging their father. Seeing them from a distance was all the comfort he needed at the end of his shift. This routine defined most of his days on COVID duty.

I also visited the district's Sadar Hospital. There, Dr R.K. mentioned that mobile vans were being sent from the district headquarters to the villages in the remotest blocks. These villages had recently started reporting cases.

I requested District Magistrate Amit Kumar to attach me to one of the mobile vans. He informed me that a mobile van was set to go to Laukahi Block, the most backward block of Madhubani, the next day.

'One of the Panchayats there has reported 16 positive cases. Would you go along with the van?' he messaged me.

I was more than willing to follow. So, I prepared for the next day. I stocked up on biscuits, chips and water bottles.

The mobile van team included thirty-seven–year–old medical officer Iftikhar Ahmad, lab technicians Santosh Kumar, twenty-nine, and Sanjay Jha, twenty-two, along with a driver. Dr R.K. was scheduled to flag off the van from Sadar Hospital. I reached Sadar, barely 500 metres from the circuit house, at 8 a.m. One of the technicians supposed to accompany the team was running late. As we waited, Dr. RK, a man in his sixties, grew increasingly annoyed and kept calling him.

Finally, after the technician arrived an hour later than planned, we set off for Jiroga Panchayat, part of Laukahi, one of the twenty-one development blocks of Madhubani district. The block spans sixty-four villages, its population is approximately 280,000. As of 21 May, it had 115 active cases and 15 containment zones.

The mobile van, named Bunyad Sanjeevni Seva (Outreach Therapy Van), was painted yellow and green and bore a poster of CM Nitish Kumar dressed in white kurta-pyjama and sporting a broad smile. Despite its large size, the van was not well-suited for the rough roads leading to Laukahi.

I followed the van in my car with Binod. After the Araria incident, he spoke little, which meant I often had to ask strangers for directions.

The journey spanned over eighty km through challenging roads, many still being built. After three days of continuous rain, the kutcha roads were muddy, and at times, it felt like we might not even reach the villages.

About fifteen km away from the Panchayat, the van got stuck on a kutcha road near a bridge under construction. Tempos were dropping passengers off on one side of the road.

Women with heavy bags on their shoulders trudged through the mud to reach the other side. Only motorcycles managed to navigate the 500-metre-long mud track.

After assessing the situation for about fifteen minutes, the team called the district headquarters to update them.

I overheard them saying they couldn't move further, the van would get stuck if it attempted to cross the dirt road.

After being rebuked by the BDO, the team decided to proceed.

Binod sat silently in the car for a while before stepping out. He walked a short distance to make some calls but couldn't due to poor signals. He continued walking until he finally got network and called the agency to inform them that he wouldn't drive on this stretch—the car would get stuck.

I was furious. The van had already left by now.

The agency called me, saying the car couldn't go further and that I should have taken a Bolero or an Innova as a Swift Dzire wasn't meant for kutcha roads.

I stood in the middle of the road under the scorching May sun.

The area barely had a phone signal. When I finally managed to reach BDO Preetam Chauhan, he immediately dispatched two bikes to my location.

I sat under a tree and waited for them to arrive.

Binod had wandered off. We eventually decided that one of the bikers would drop me off at the village, while Binod would follow the other biker, taking a longer, motorable route there. Luckily, the van and I arrived in the village around the same time. The van was parked outside Jiroga panchayat's middle school campus, which was waterlogged from recent rain.

The mobile van team had 400 RAT (Rapid Antigen Test) kits. As they prepared for the villagers to arrive, one lab technician donned a PPE kit while the other arranged chairs and set out the kits on the desk. Meanwhile, the doctor sat down with a register, and some ASHA workers sat down in the corridor.

Medical officer Iftikhar Ahmad was ready to launch the testing camp. They waited. And they waited. And they waited. No one turned up.

Some villagers lingered on the fringes of the school, peering in into the campus.

The school had been closed for the past year and a half. Wild grass and insects had overtaken the old building. A herd of goats was grazing nearby. While we waited, I asked the Anganwadi workers to call the village head, so he could help convince the villagers to get tested.

Half an hour passed, no villagers showed up. When the village head finally arrived, three ASHA workers, Kamini Devi (forty),

Savitri Devi (forty-two), Ekavari Devi (thirty-eight), accompanied by their husbands, decided to make another round of the village. I joined them to understand why the villagers were reluctant to get tested.

They refused to get tested for various reasons. Some made lame excuses, some argued with the ASHA workers and others accused them of being paid to spread Coronavirus.

The door-to-door campaign lasted all of thirty minutes, and we returned, defeated.

BDO Preetam Chauhan had informed the village head Shravan Kumar and the local ASHA workers about the testing drive a day before the camp.

The ASHA workers had gone door-to-door to inform the villagers. By the time the van arrived, they had already done two rounds. The village head had also urged people to come forward for testing. Despite these efforts, the turnout was minimal.

Meanwhile, Ahmad noticed some people still lingering at the school boundary, and it was no less than a ray of hope. He decided to get himself tested.'Mera kar do test, woh dekhenge toh shayad kara lenge,' he told the lab technicians. (Do my test, maybe then they'll come forward.) But nobody crossed the boundary line.

Then, the three ASHA workers' husbands volunteered to get tested.

The situation was very similar to the film *Newton*, where Rajkumar Rao's character waits for hours with his polling team for the tribals to come and cast their vote. Each member of the testing team looked anxious and restless, but I also saw determination in their eyes.

An hour and a half later, only four tests had been completed—all of them of the team members. All negative.

The doctor then walked towards the crowd lingering outside the school campus.

'See, four people have been tested and the results are negative. Please come forward. I assure you that nothing will happen to you even if you test positive.' Despite his reassurance, many recoiled in fear.

The doctor returned to his chair, and I decided to approach the villagers.

A migrant worker said the testing team might be COVID carriers. I insisted that they get tested, sharing that I had been tested in various districts without any issues.

Other villagers began to speak up, revealing their fears that a positive diagnosis would be a death sentence. They shared horror stories, believing those who tested positive would be taken to a distant building and left to die.

This fear was fuelled by last year's experiences when returning migrant workers were quarantined in decrepit buildings.

'Pichhle saal inhone school mein saanp-bichchhuon ke saath chhod diya tha. Kyon test karayein? Test positive aane ka matlab hai ki ya hospital le jaakar maar denge ya fir sarkari school mein,' said forty-four-year-old Suresh Kumar Yadav. (Last year, they left people in old school buildings teeming with snakes and scorpions. Why should we get tested? A positive diagnosis means you'll be left to die either in a hospital or a government school.)

Among the villagers peering in from the school boundary, some were coughing. I asked if anyone in the village had had a fever, cough, chest pain or breathing problems in recent days.

Most admitted that the village was suffering from COVID-like symptoms, but their sources of information—on 'hacks' and medication to beat COVID—were YouTube or other social media platforms. They were 'drinking hot water and eating spicy food' to prevent or treat symptoms. Many added that they relied on village quacks for treatment, who charged 150 rupees for medicines.

'Bhaap lene se theek ho jata hai. Maine dekha tha YouTube par. Yeh mask mein kitaanu hote hain jisse virus failta hai. Isliye gamchha lagana chahiye.' (Inhaling steam cures it. I saw it on YouTube. These masks contain germs that spread the virus. That's why we should use a gamchha instead.)

The mobile van team members joined in to help me convince the villagers.

A twenty-eight-year-old migrant worker, Sunil Yadav, who had returned to the village during the previous year's lockdown, retorted, 'Khud toh ye kavach pehen kar aaye ho, sau logon ka testing karke humko Corona failaaoge. Hum kyon karayein testing? Tum log baahar se aaye ho, tumko Corona hua toh?' (You're wearing this protective gear. You will test a hundred people and spread COVID. Why should we get tested? You people have travelled from another place, what if you have the disease?)

After several futile attempts, the doctor returned to his desk.

The village head then requested his aides to get tested. Although initially reluctant, they eventually agreed. An ASHA worker also stepped forward.

Over the next two hours, these were the only tests conducted.

Towards the end, two young men approached me, mentioning that they had a fever, and asked if they should get tested, and their results, like the others, were negative.

By 3.30 p.m., when it was time to wrap up, only nine people had been tested in the village of approximately 2,800 residents. Of these, seven were from the testing team and the district and village administration. Deflated and exhausted, the team prepared for the four-hour journey back to district headquarters.

Later that day, I detailed the situation on the ground to District Magistrate Amit Kumar. One of his proposed solutions was to use social media—the very source of misinformation—to combat it. 'I have decided to tackle this misinformation by engaging influential Mithila people. We will ask them to make two-minute videos about testing and the stigma attached to COVID. Apart from that, we will also start publicity campaigns in remote blocks to inform people that even if someone tests positive, they won't be taken anywhere.' He had a third strategy as well. 'We will ask PDS dealers, who provide ration in villages, to counter this fear and misinformation since they interact regularly with most of the villagers.'

This strategy worked—not just for COVID testing but vaccination as well.

During the second wave, shrouds became a symbol of the devastation the pandemic wreaked, especially in the rural areas of Uttar Pradesh and Bihar. Photographs of shallow mass graves with bodies covered in kafans along the banks of the Ganga shook India's conscience. During the peak of the wave, the absence of transparent death statistics left the dead to tell their own stories.

Even now, transparency around COVID death statistics remains elusive.

After Binod refused to drive me, I had to return to Patna. The travel agency had sent a new driver, Chhotu Mishra. Contrary to what his name might suggest, Mishra was a tall man in his late forties. He spoke little and constantly chewed gutka. And he knew his way around the state.

The agency had informed him that he would only be accompanying me for a week.

I called an old friend from my Delhi University days. Over lunch at her home in Patna, we discussed the challenging situation in rural Bihar.

At five that evening, I started for Gaya.

We entered Gaya in the late evening hours. The once touristy, vibrant city now looked deserted. Tourist buses were parked at bus stands and private lots. Roadside eateries were closed.

Locals who ran shops in front of monasteries played cards to pass the time. The monasteries that had distributed ration and relief packages during the first wave had run out of supplies. The hotel where I intended to check in had been shut for months with no staff in sight. It had been booked online by my office in Delhi.

'WiFi?' I inquired at the reception.

'Madam, band padaa hai. Abhi check karna padega,' the man said as he went upstairs. Since it didn't seem like he'd come back any time soon, I decided to look for other places where I could find basic facilities like food and WiFi. I needed a good internet connection to send my stories to New Delhi.

After taking a round of the city, we found an old hotel called The Royal Residency near the Mahabodhi Temple in Bodh Gaya. Chhotu had been here before with other travellers.

We were in the last week of May and the rains were relentless, so I couldn't venture into the rural areas. Later in the evening, I visited the COVID hospitals, crematoriums and the primary health centre. The number of patients had started to decline, there were no queues at crematoriums, and pharmacies also saw fewer people coming in for medicines like paracetamol.

The second wave in India peaked in early May 2021. By mid-May, the number of new cases began to decline. By the end of May, the situation had improved considerably, with a notable reduction in both new cases and fatalities.

On 26 May, India reported 26,948,874 confirmed cases and 307,231 deaths. After reaching a peak of 414,188 daily cases on 7 May, there was a continuous decline in new infections. By 26 May, the number of new cases had dropped to 19,235 per million.[1]

According to statistics from the World Health Organisation (WHO), during the week of 16 May to 22 May 2022, over 3.7 million cases were reported worldwide, marking a 3 per cent decrease compared to the previous week. The number of new weekly deaths also declined, with over 9,000 reported deaths, recording an 11 per cent decrease from the previous week.[2]

I bought newspapers from the previous days to understand what had been happening as the dust began to settle. In one of the local newspapers, I came across a short article about the weavers of Patwa Toli. The town is home to about 150 traditional weavers' families, primarily from the Patwa community. During the second wave, the weavers' business saw an unexpected boom due to the rising demand for kafans, the saffron shrouds used in funeral rites.

Patwatoli, a small town located in Gaya district's Manpur block, situated on the banks of the Phalgu river, is renowned for its handloom industry.

The Phalgu river is an important one for the Hindus. It is estimated that around 8 lakh pilgrims visit the Phalgu river every year during Pitru Paksha to perform Pind Daan to seek salvation for deceased ancestors.

But the sacred river does not flow all year round, it is a monsoon river. For most of the year, the water remains beneath the surface, and what's visible is a vast expanse of sand dunes. According to a popular legend, this is due to a curse by Goddess Sita.

Given that Gaya is a drought-prone district and the river is not a major source of water for the locals, Nitish Kumar initiated an ambitious project to bring the Ganga's water to Gaya—one of the most successful initiatives of his tenure. To rejuvenate the Phalgu, Nitish Kumar allocated a budget of ₹324 crore for the construction of Gayaji Dam.

The Gayaji Dam, India's longest river dam, was under construction when I visited the site in May 2021. On 8 September 2022, more than a year later, Nitish Kumar inaugurated the dam along with a steel foot overbridge.

Apart from being a handloom hub, Patwatoli has, over the years, gained fame for producing the highest number of IITians, earning it the media label of 'IIT Village'.[3]

In no time, Chhotu and I were walking in the narrow lanes of Patwatoli. The sound of looms came from every house. The town barely slept in those days.

I met fifty-year-old Jitendra Prasad at his three-storey home where swathes of saffron shrouds were hung out to dry on his terrace. The other congested floors were filled with raw materials, and nine power looms ran non-stop to meet the high demand for shrouds.

Prasad admitted that business was booming. Not only were his nine power looms operating eighteen hours a day, but he also had had to rent additional machines. 'I had to rent nine more looms last month as the demand for kafans has increased drastically. It is three times higher than my usual sales,' Prasad told me

He added, 'We've been overworked this month. Our labourers had fled due to fear of COVID initially, but now we've had to call them back because we couldn't manage without them.'

According to Prasad, he sold over 40,000 kafans in April alone. For a weaver like him, these massive sales were unprecedented.

'On average, we sell 25,000 kafans in the summer months. Last year, due to the first lockdown, sales dropped by 40 per cent, but things are different in the second wave,' Prasad said.

His family had been weaving kafans for the last twenty years. 80 per cent of their products were sold in Bihar and the remaining were sent to West Bengal and Jharkhand.

Prasad, fifty, confessed that he sometimes grappled with the dilemma of how one should feel about this surge in demand, especially since his eighty-year-old father had succumbed to the virus on 28 April.

After the death, Prasad had shut his machines for two weeks.

'Lekin itna zyada demand tha ki phir kaam chaalu karna pada. Kharab toh lagta hi hai lekin hum nahin banayenge toh kaun banaayega?' he said. (I had to restart work as the demand increased. Of course, we feel terrible about the deaths, but what other option do we have? It is our profession to make kafans.)

I met more weavers and locals involved in the business of kafans. The residents in the area told me that they were worried as over a hundred people had tested positive in the second wave and 15 had died in Patwatoli alone.

This was giving them nightmares. But for some families, making kafans became the sole source of income when other means of livelihood were scarce.

There were twenty weavers like Prasad in the town who manufactured kafans.

Among the biggest was Paras Nath, with thirty-five power looms of his own.

'I produce 400 kafans a day, and my stock sells out daily now,' he said. 'Earlier, we had to stockpile the kafans; there were fewer deaths during the summer.'

Kafans made by Prasad and Nath were sold for Rs 10 and Rs 30, respectively. (The price was decided by the size and quality of the cloth used.)

Durgeshwar Prasad, a weaver who had led me to Prasad's house, told me, 'I make kafans along with gamchhas. At this time, selling shrouds has helped keep my business afloat. With trains not running and rural markets on hold, gamchha sales have declined. Without the sound of the looms, we can't sleep at night. This is our livelihood. Last year, the lockdown hit us hard, but now selling kafans is helping us survive. We dread this pandemic, but we have to meet the demand to ensure dignity in death.'[4]

I thought digging some more might throw some light on the gap between official statistics and the actual number of COVID deaths. I spoke to various middlemen, shopkeepers and retailers.

Most people were afraid to speak to the media, afraid that revealing their identities would lead to trouble. The government had been booking journalists for arranging oxygen cylinders for dying patients.

But I managed to speak with a few individuals. Only Prem Bhagat, a retailer from Hajipur district who sourced his materials from Patwatoli, agreed to go on record. He said that he had ordered over 40,000 kafans in April and May to sell to cremation ghats in Patna and the surrounding districts.

'This is not a regular year. The demand has been unprecedented,' he told me.

'Villages are buying in bulk. This wasn't the case in the first wave when our business suffered.'

After filing the story, I left for my next destination—Rohtas. It was going to be a four-hour journey through heavy rain.

On our way, we passed through Aurangabad district. I had been on the road for over fifty days. As I was crossing Sone Diara, I saw huge cranes in the distance. They were digging sand. Even amidst a raging pandemic, the illegal sand miners continued their operations. The Sone river has been severely exploited by the sand mafia. A toxic nexus of police, politicians and businessmen mines the Sone and the Ganga. Gang wars over sand are common in the state.

In Rohtas, I stayed in the district headquarters, Sasaram.

There was much discussion on social media about the Bhoj ceremonies (funeral feasts) following COVID-19 deaths. Some viewed these ceremonies as vulgar, noting that poor families, unable to afford treatment, were forced into debt to organise these local feasts. Others believed that the deceased, often deprived of dignity during their last rites, deserved this final act of respect.

On one hand, Bhoj ceremonies were elaborate and drew huge crowds but they were also intimate community affairs where journalists were nosy outsiders.

I realised that getting details or attending a shradh as a reporter would be challenging. People usually allow a reporter to become a part of their lives, but death in the pandemic was not just personal, it was political.

So, I turned to BDOs to ask about Bhoj across villages, assuming they might have a list of permissions for large gatherings. However, they were unaware of any such permissions.

Without local assistance, I decided to venture into villages, randomly asking people if there were any upcoming Bhoj ceremonies. In one of the blocks, I stopped in a village where three weddings were taking place, with large gatherings in attendance. Haryana's pop queen Sapna Chaudhary's songs were blaring from loudspeakers, and young men and women dressed in bright clothes were dancing to the tunes.

I got down from the car to speak to the crowd. Most people were unapologetic. They had already postponed the weddings for a year, and the girls weren't getting any younger. Plus it was much cheaper to hold weddings during the pandemic.

I ventured deeper into the hinterlands, to find a family organising a Bhoj. In Baraon village of Nokha block, I finally found a family preparing for a feast for eighty-five-year-old Urmila Devi, who had died of COVID a fortnight ago.

A local friend agreed to accompany me that day. Being from the area, he managed to convince the family to speak with me.

'This time, there won't be a crowd, just a few neighbours will come for the bhoj,' said Uma Shankar Singh, a neighbour and relative of late Urmila Devi. Uma Shankar, along with a few relatives and priests, was preparing for the puja before the feast. They initially mistook me for a district official and explained that they had not sought permission but felt obligated to organise the event.

'Otherwise, people will boycott us in social gatherings. We have to do this,' he pleaded, trying to convince me.

Despite Uma Shankar's belief that not many would attend, a crowd of 600 turned up for Urmila Devi's shradh bhoj on the 13th day of her death.

Uma Shankar's expectation of a small turnout was not unfounded. The fear of COVID was all pervasive by now. The same fear and stigma as in the case of the Araria orphans could be felt here. Urmila's family had done their best to hide the cause of her death.

'I was worried when my mother showed symptoms,' said her youngest son, fifty-nine-year-old Amarender Singh.

After having delayed getting her tested, when the results finally confirmed she had COVID, the family kept it a secret and did not take her to a hospital. Despite their efforts, word went around.

Ajay Kumar, a resident of the village, told me, 'These days if someone falls sick, people immediately think—what if it's Corona. So they avoid going to that person's house. And she (Urmila Devi) had all the symptoms of the disease.'

Her funeral on 21 May 2021 was attended by only a dozen close relatives, which the village residents said was the usual practice even before the pandemic. However, the Bhoj was a different matter. A Bhoj is usually attended by the entire village. Late Urmila Devi's family members and neighbours said that 600 attendees for her Bhoj was a modest number; in pre-COVID times, there would have been over 1,000 guests.[5]

Feasting for the COVID dead felt vulgar to me. Many of the deceased were denied the medical care they deserved. Most deaths resulted from delayed testing, lack of hospital beds and misinformation about the disease.

In village after village, as I travelled through rural Bihar, I observed that while the fear of infection had stigmatised COVID to the extent that families often hid cases or mourned deaths alone, weddings and funeral feasts or Bhoj, continued to draw hundreds of people—without masks or adherence to social distancing norms.

'When we eat at the feasts organised by other families, we too must invite others when there is a death in our family. It's customary. If someone doesn't do it, they will be alienated by the village. So the Bhoj has to be organised, even if one has to sell their house or land to feed others,' a guest at Urmila Devi's Bhoj underlined its role within the rural society.

He stressed that adherence to customs was paramount, regardless of the cause of death.

'It doesn't matter if the deceased was a COVID patient. The family will have to organise a feast and invite others. Those who are scared will not come. Others will.'

According to the Bihar state government figures, there had been 5,163 COVID deaths in the state by the first week of June 2021. This would imply a near-equal number of Bhoj gatherings.

Urmila Devi's family spent approximately 2 lakhs on feeding neighbours and relatives.

When I asked about the cost of her treatment, a family member replied that they had spent only Rs 12,000.

Two days before the Bhoj, another ritual, the shradh, was organised. A 'small' feast was prepared for more than 200 people.

Urmila Devi's son Amarender Singh said, 'Bhoj to karna hi padega. (We have to organise a Bhoj.) We can't upset people, can we?'

Meanwhile, some family members were still trying to assure everyone who had attended the smaller feast that Urmila Devi hadn't died of COVID.

'If she was COVID-positive, then why didn't any of us get it from her? Ten of us live under the same roof. We looked after her,' one of her grandsons, Ajit, tried to placate the guests.

Every ancestor of the Singh family had been cremated at the Manikarnika Ghat in Varanasi, but the pandemic disrupted this tradition. Some of Urmila's daughters, who lived in distant metro cities, couldn't travel to attend her funeral. She was cremated in the village crematorium. The family worried that the departed soul wouldn't find peace.

In the Mahadalit tolas in Rohtas district, people talked about distant relatives who had died, apparently, after receiving the vaccine.

In the media, discussions about a potential third wave had already begun. By extension, the spotlight fell on communities that were lagging behind in the vaccination drive.

The pandemic was exposing the country's significant digital divide, as remote areas struggled to keep up with the central government's web-based vaccination campaign. This had to be my next story.

I visited one of Bihar's remotest and least populated blocks, Adhaura, fifty-eight km from the well-connected district headquarters in Kaimur.

When I discussed the idea with a friend in the bureaucracy, he joked, 'Your Bihar trip is complete now. We haven't even seen that block. It is considered a punishment post for BDOs.' In the bureaucracy, underdeveloped districts are often considered punishment postings.

This conversation reminded me of an excerpt from the book *Life in the IAS: My Encounters with the Three Lals of Haryana* by former IAS officer Ram Verma. In his seminal work on Haryana politics, Verma vividly described how, in the 1970s, IAS officers were sent to the Narnaul-Mahendragarh area as a 'punishment posting'. For decades, Mahendragarh, my home district, was disparaged as the second Kalapani by Haryana's bureaucracy. Mahendragarh was once known for its broken roads and arid landscape.

In his book, Ram Verma wrote that the journey from Rohtak to south and northwestern Haryana was marked by a bumpy ride on 'raw unkempt roads' and the sight of women travelling far to fetch water, with children in their arms.

Residents of backward and underdeveloped districts often believe they are the most disadvantaged in terms of human development indicators. Until they see places like Adhaura, they might not realise the extent of their own relative progress. It becomes challenging to determine which block is worse off. Places like Adhaura stand out because they lack even basic infrastructure like mobile towers.[6]

Reporting from the block, or even reaching it, would have been impossible without a local contact. Someone in the administration connected me with Vishwanath Pahadia, a tribal man with roots in the block. He was a social worker active in the area. For outreach initiatives in the tribal belt, the district administrations had enlisted the help of activists like him.

He agreed to accompany me. Before the trip, he cautioned me about heavy rains, warning that the car might get stuck for days.

However, when I called him one day before my visit, he sounded non-committal, so I decided to go on my own. The next morning, at 7 a.m., I received a call from an upset Pahadia because I hadn't sent the car to pick him up yet. I sensed that my temperament might not sit well with him. Nevertheless, I sent the car. Unsure if we would find food later in the day, we had breakfast together.

Pahadia was visibly impatient about everything, constantly hustling, always on the move.

As we entered the hilly block, the driver stopped to offer prayers at the Mushar temple, a significant local landmark in the block. Drivers and travellers stop to offer prayers to the deity here, believing that failing to offer a beedi and matchbox could lead to unfortunate road accidents. Chhotu Mishra, my driver, too got down to buy a matchbox and a beedi bundle from a nearby shop.

I noticed that every passerby, whether on a bus, tractor or bike, was stopping at the entrance before going further.

The road to the block had been recently constructed. Pahadia had been calling his relatives in the block, telling everyone that a big car was coming and they should all come and see.

He later explained that since the area lacked a mobile tower and people had to climb down the hill to make calls, seeing a car would be a big deal for the children. He also wanted to impress his relatives by showing that since moving to an urban area, he had become important enough to travel by car.

On our way to the block office, we passed through many villages where Pahadia would stop and call out to the villagers.

'Ae adiwasi, idhar aao.' (Hey tribal, come here!)

At one point, I objected. He was a tribal himself—why was he intimidating other tribals or demeaning them? Pahadia had an explanation.

He said that if he spoke softly, the villagers wouldn't take us seriously. So, we should pretend to be important people.

By this time, the Bihar government had launched the Home Isolation Tracking (HIT) app, designed to monitor COVID-19 patients across the state. The app was receiving extensive coverage in newspapers.

But in Adhaura, forget about accessing central government's COWIN app, very few had even heard of the state's HIT app.

So the district administration wasn't tackling just vaccine hesitancy but also the delay in dissemination of other COVID-relation information due to poor internet connectivity.

When we arrived at the BDO's office, he was out in the field. We waited for half an hour. The evening before, I had spoken with Kaimur's deputy development commissioner, Kumar Gaurav, who had sent a message to the BDO, Alok Kumar Sharma, informing him of my visit.

Sharma received that message right in front of us, over twenty-four hours later. Sharma, a thirty-year-old BPSC (Bihar Public Service Commission) passed officer, explained the lengths his team had to go to just to send a WhatsApp message to the Kaimur headquarters.

'A team member travels 22 km to a point on the Uttar Pradesh border where he gets connectivity. From there, he sends messages to the headquarters. To send one message, I need a man, a bike, and petrol to cover 22 km,' he explained while pouring Pahadia, the driver and me tea in his office.

Sharma was posted in another district earlier.

'This is considered a punishment post. There's nothing here. Many times, BDOs are posted only on paper and don't even report for duty,' he said.

His helplessness was evident as he spoke about the lack of resources in this remote block, a tribal area cut off from the world.

The 118 villages here were surrounded by forests and had a population of 57,000. More than six panchayats here had not seen a road yet. During monsoon, these villages became completely inaccessible to the district administration.

But the silver lining was that the block was declared COVID free on 23 May. Cases were mild, and not a single patient had required hospitalisation, the BDO told me. But inaccessibility was a significant challenge to the vaccination drive in this case. Only 2,000 people had received the first dose when I visited the area on 30 May.

Rumours didn't need the internet to spread here; they travelled the old-fashioned way—by word of mouth and hearsay.

The vaccination drive had been working fine before misleading stories started circulating.

BDO Sharma said, 'I feel so frustrated now. Not a single villager can be convinced to take the vaccine because misinformation spreads rapidly.'

A significant portion of the 1,000 doses delivered to Adhaura on 13 May remained unused.

Not a single shot had been administered on the weekend before my visit, prompting Sharma to discuss the issue with police and local politicians. Convincing tribes like the Korvas, who lived on the jungle's periphery, proved to be the most challenging for him.

'They won't come to the village panchayat or the block office to get vaccinated. We have to chase after them. With the monsoon approaching, our work will become even more difficult. And I believe a third wave is coming too,' he was apprehensive.

In the block, 80 per cent of the tribal population belonged to the Kharwars, 4 per cent to the Chero and 13 per cent to the Agadiya. The administration actively engaged with community leaders, family heads, village chiefs and government representatives to ensure that people were persuaded to get vaccinated. Once one family received the dose, others followed their example. At times, the community head had to sit among the people and personally demonstrate that a single dose of the vaccine wasn't a death warrant. It took extensive efforts from all involved to finally vaccinate the entire block.

I recounted to the BDO how some tribals had mistaken me for a government official there to vaccinate them and fled to the jungles, fearing forced vaccination when my car stopped at their villages on my way to the headquarters.

As I travelled from one village to another, the stories of people 'dying from the vaccine' became increasingly intriguing.

About twenty km from the block office was Karar village, home to forty-five-year-old Malti Chero Chaudhary. She was very wary of strangers. When she saw us parking our car, she ran inside her house and hid for a while.

After some time, she came out to ask if the vaccination programme was a 'conspiracy to kill us'.

'I heard three people died in Hathini after taking the shot,' she said.

Things were not very different in Bardeeha village. The elderly were fearful of the vaccine. Some who had received the first dose a month ago were dreading the second, since one man in the village experienced a mild fever that lasted several days. But while many complained that the vaccine could be fatal, twenty-five-year-old Saurabh Kumar expressed his desire to get vaccinated.

He asked me to record his statement. Standing outside a mud-plastered house with a bicycle hanging on its front wall, I began recording him. The first thing he highlighted was the story of internet deprivation in the age of TikTok. Then he addressed the issue of the vaccines. 'Yahan log ghabraaye hue hain ki lagwate hi mar jayenge. Lekin humko toh lagwana hai. Pata chal nahin paa raha hai kab lag raha hai. Gaadi nahin hai toh jile ya block mein nahin ja sakte.' (People fear that vaccine may instantly kill them. But I want to take it. I don't know where the centre is and I don't have a vehicle to visit the district or block headquarters.)

When I asked if he knew about the COWIN or HIT apps, he said he hadn't heard of them.

He said he had to travel three km from his home to find a spot with mobile network.

'There is no WhatsApp or YouTube here, so we get information from TV,' he said.

After spending a day in the block and being cut off from the internet myself, I left the Adhaura block that evening, feeling a bit relieved to have my Twitter, WhatsApp and Instagram back.

DDC Kumar Gaurav highlighted that a letter had already been sent to the state government to take the vaccination drive offline in these remote areas.

Pahadia was a little upset because we had missed visiting a few villages that he wanted to see. He had already boasted to his relatives that he, along with the journalist, was going to meet the CM to discuss their issues. I had never made such a claim to him.

The next morning, … Pahadia called me and rattled off a long list of grievances against the government. I clarified that the CM's office was unaware of the situation and that the best I could do was connect him to the Collector at Kaimur. Pahadia wasn't impressed.

It wasn't just blocks like Adhaura which were facing massive resistance to vaccination; marginalised castes living in mainstream areas were also rejecting the vaccine.

On 31 May, I accompanied a vaccination team comprising the BDO, ANMs (Auxiliary Nurse Midwife[7]) and ASHA workers to Amarpur tola in Nawada district to report on vaccine hesitancy among the Mahadalits.

Upon seeing the team, nearly half the people fled to the fields and disappeared. A few village representatives were sent to call them back, but they did not return. Some women and children had stayed behind to look after the cattle and households. They did not come out when the ASHA workers called them.

The team was led by forty-seven-year-old Mahendra Manjhi, the husband of ASHA worker Dhanno Devi. Manjhi was among the fifteen people vaccinated on 26 May during a vaccination camp in the village. The district administration had chosen Manjhi as a poster boy to motivate the tola.

Of the fifteen, eight were women and seven men. Most men were from the families of either ASHA workers or ANMs, ordinary people were not getting vaccinated at all.

Amarpur Musahari, a Mahadalit tola, was part of the Kharant panchayat in Nawada Sadar block with approximately 160 households. Kharant panchayat, with a population of 5,294, includes nine Mahadalit tolas.

Mahadalits are the poorest social groups within the Dalit community, making up around 15 per cent of Bihar's population—there were 1,539 Mahadalit tolas in Nawada district alone. Up until the 2011 caste census, the population of Mahadalits in Nawada was 141,949.

When the vaccination team reached the house of thirty-five-year-old Lalita Devi, a Mahadalit, she shooed them away. Lalita's objection: the government wasn't paying people to take the vaccine.

'Lockdown laga deve toh sarkar humari ka ek rupaiya deve? Suiya le leve to sarkar humri ka ek rupaiya deve? Ee maati ka ghar hai, din raat kamave ke suiya leve? Kaahe leve suiya?' (The government announced a lockdown but didnt give us a penny. Now it wants us to get this vaccine. But it still won't give us a penny. I live in this kutcha house. We work day and night to earn our daily bread. Should we skip work to get this vaccine?)

Nearly everyone in Amarpur Musahari was asking the same question: Why should they take the vaccine without any monetary incentive?

Chhotu, my driver, made an interesting observation: 'Madam, media ka sunkar abhi mask baanta gaya hai.' (Madam, they have only just now started distributing masks to the villagers because they were told someone from the media was coming.)

He was right. Everyone had surgical masks hanging below their noses.

Fifty-four-year-old ANM Rani Urmila said, 'They believe that Corona is an "AC disease" that will never reach the working class. They question why the government is giving them a free vaccine, what the motive behind it is.'

'We are sending teams, but no one turns up,' BDO Kumar Shailendra said.

Despite these challenges, the vaccination drive was progressing on the ground, albeit very slowly. (Ten days after my visit to the village, I called ANM Rani Urmila who informed me that only nine more people had got the jab, bringing the total to twenty-four in the tola.)

Interestingly, Chintu (name changed to protect identity), a Dom from Rohtas district, compared the vaccination drive to elections.

'They give us money during elections. Why not support us now with the free vaccine when we are unemployed in this lockdown?' he asked me, suggesting that free ration or even a couple of 100 rupees along with the vaccine would help.

Standing next to him, his wife added, 'We belong to the lowest of all castes. The government should talk to us and provide some benefits along with the vaccine.'

In Amarpur Musahari, I met Ajay Manjhi, who was returning home from work. He called himself Ajay Devgan.

'If we get infected, we will look to God, not the government, for help. Even if we are on the brink of death due to Coronavirus, we won't take the vaccine,' he said.

I spoke to several district magistrates. One, speaking on the condition of anonymity, said:

> We have always successfully implemented women and child-centric welfare schemes through ASHA workers and ANMs. This workforce has been most effective until now. But this time, men need to be convinced, and ASHA workers are facing a lot of hostility.
>
> There are many reasons behind this. First, there is a lot of misinformation across castes and classes. However, the poorest communities among Dalits and religious groups are more rigid. Secondly, there is a monetary benefit angle to this.

His administration planned to enlist the help of Vikas Mitras and PDS dealers, who have a strong influence in their communities.

In the coming months, stories emerged from many states where citizens were told they had to get vaccinated or risk losing access to welfare schemes. This approach worked in some cases.

Speaking about this approach, Nawada's district magistrate, Yashpal Meena said, 'We will select a few role models in the tolas. These individuals will then motivate others to get vaccinated.'

He also shared data which showed the curve of vaccination rising day by day. On 1 June, Nawada vaccinated 605 people. On 10 June, the district vaccinated 3,725 people, including 3,660 who received their first dose and sixty-five who received their second dose.

The Mahadalit tolas were still reporting lower numbers. 'Due to lower literacy rates in these areas, the vaccination drive is going slower compared to other areas,' Meena explained.

According to him, senior administrative officers at the district, sub-division and block levels were also visiting areas with lower vaccination rates, especially the Mahadalit tolas, to motivate people, address their concerns and dispel rumours.

The administration also started sending the vaccination mobile vans to Mahadalit tolas and panchayats to make it more convenient for people to get vaccinated.

'Is this helping?' I asked Meena.

'I've seen signs of progress in the last ten days,' he said.

My driver, Chhotu Mishra, too, was hesitating to get vaccinated. 'Humare Bihar mein na madam, nakli vaccine ban gaya hoga. Dus din ke bheetar ban jata hai. Hum zindagi mein kabhi nahin lagwayenge.' (In our Bihar, madam, a fake vaccine must have been made by now. It takes just ten days. I will never get vaccinated.)

Despite these challenges, India's vaccination campaign is considered to be one of the most successful vaccination campaigns in terms of scale and efficiency.

By October 2021, India had administered over 100 crore doses in less than nine months, reported *The Indian Express*.[8]

According to a PIB (Press Information Bureau) press release, as of 6 January 2023, India had administered more than 220 crore COVID-19 vaccine doses across the country.[9] Ninety-seven per cent of eligible beneficiaries had received at least one dose, and around 90 per cent had received both doses. In short, India managed to vaccinate a significant portion of its population in a relatively short time.

Additionally, India exported vaccines to nearly a hundred countries, demonstrating its capacity to produce and distribute vaccines on a global scale.[10]

After Nawada, we headed to Bhagalpur, crossing Jamui and Munger districts. I stayed in Bhagalpur for two days. By this time, the administration's focus had shifted away from the queues at hospitals and crematoriums. District Magistrate Subrat Kumar Sen mentioned that he was focusing on setting up a new oxygen plant.

The vaccination story, which was also my final piece on COVID coverage, was published in the second week of June. By then, I had returned to Delhi.

Before leaving for Delhi, my home, Chhotu Mishra and I indulged in some shopping. We stopped at a local market and bought Jardalu mangoes which Bagalpur is famous for. I bought five kilos for myself, and Chhotu ended up buying forty kilos. His daughter, a twelfth grader, kept calling him throughout the journey. He would speak very affectionately, promising to return soon. I had grown fond of him. We were like co-travellers on an arduous journey in the time of COVID.

Our car was redolent with the fragrance of mangoes as we set off for our very final trip to Kishanganj district. As we crossed the mighty Kosi river, I asked Chhotu to pull over. I needed a moment to myself.

My assignment was coming to an end. I had tears in my eyes. I looked back on the roads taken, the scenes of devastation and the ravaged faces I had met along the way over a span of sixty days. Just a few days into the travels, I had started wanting to finish the assignment and return home. Yet the thought of this journey coming to an end now filled me with a strange sorrow.

Chhotu, too, became emotional on the day of our departure. We had been companions for the last fifteen days. His happy-go-lucky attitude and sense of humour had made the final leg of my assignment memorable. That's how I will always remember him. Though I do hope he has taken the vaccine by now. And I certainly look forward to crossing paths with him again.

Notes

PROLOGUE

1. PTI, The Hindu, 'Coronavirus |COVID-19 is not health emergency, no need to panic: Health Ministry', (https://www.thehindu.com/news/national/coronavirus-outbreak-union-health-ministry-press-conference-in-new-delhi/article31061163.ece)
2. Yadav, Jyoti, 'Skill ministry employee claims his mother is COVID 19-positive, later says it was a rumour', (https://theprint.in/india/skill-ministry-employee-claims-his-mother-is-covid-19-positive-later-says-it-was-a-rumour/383519/)
3. The Hindu desk, 'Coronavirus updates | March 20, 2020', (https://www.thehindu.com/news/national/coronavirus-live-updates-march-20-2020/article31115014.ece)
4. Chappell, Bill , 'Coronavirus: 100,000 More Cases Reported Worldwide In Less Than 2 Weeks'. (https://www.npr.org/sections/coronavirus-live-updates/2020/03/20/818853368/coronavirus-infected-100-000-more-people-worldwide-in-less-than-2-weeks)
5. The wire staff, 'Coronavirus Updates, March 19: India Reports 4th Death, Bars International Commercial Flights', (https://science.thewire.in/health/coronavirus-updates-march-19-covid-19-sars-cov-2/)
6. Prime Minister's Office, 'PM calls for complete lockdown of entire nation for 21 days', (https://www.pib.gov.in/PressReleasePage.aspx?PRID=1608009)
7. S, Rukmini, 'India had one of the world's strictest lockdowns. Why are cases still rising?', (https://www.theguardian.com/commentisfree/2020/jul/04/india-lockdowns-cases-rising-)

1. A LONG WAY FROM HOME

1. Yadav, Jyoti, 'Highways are now paths for buffaloes, migrants cycling back home as lockdown continues', (https://theprint.in/in-pictures/highways-are-now-paths-for-buffaloes-migrants-cycling-back-home-as-lockdown-continues/416142/)
2. Taskin, Bismee, Yadav, Jyoti, 'UP's Rampur villages show signs of Covid impact: Milk sales down, shops selling on credit', (https://theprint.in/india/ups-rampur-villages-show-signs-of-covid-impact-milk-sales-down-shops-selling-on-credit/417024/)
3. Ministry of Railways, Government of India, 'Subject: Movement of Stranded Persons by Shramik Special Trains' (https://prsindia.org/files/covid19/notifications/4429.IND_Rail_Details%20Shramik%20Special%20Trains_May_02.pdf)
4. Gandhi, Rahul, (https://x.com/RahulGandhi/status/1257149860374962177)
5. Special correspondent, 'Congress will pay for rail travel of migrant workers, says Sonia Gandhi', (https://www.thehindu.com/news/national/congress-will-pay-for-rail-travel-of-migrant-workers-says-sonia-gandhi/article31497707.ece0)
6. Sensharma, Aalok, 'Centre paying 85% expenses of Shramik Special Trains, states only giving 15% fares: Railways', (https://www.thedailyjagran.com/india/centre-paying-85-per-cent-expenses-of-shramik-special-trains-states-only-giving-15-per-cent-fares-railways-10012166)
7. Patra, Sambit, (https://x.com/sambitswaraj/status/1257156770386055170)
8. Dhingra, Sanya, 'Modi govt finally clarifies it's not paying Shramik Express fare, says states footing bill', (https://theprint.in/india/governance/modi-govt-finally-clarifies-its-not-paying-shramik-express-fare-says-states-footing-bill/431410/)
9. Krar, Parshant, 'Punjab registers over 6.4 lakh migrant workers keen to return to native states', (https://economictimes.indiatimes.com/news/politics-and-nation/punjab-registers-over-6-4-lakh-migrant-workers-keen-to-return-to-native-states/articleshow/75521039.cms)
10. Sidhu, KBS, former IAS, (https://x.com/kbssidhu1961/status/1257673753137303558?s=46&t=KPQapKrfYox4I1p ZT09_0A)
11. Department of Good Governance and Information Technology,

Punjab, (https://dit.punjab.gov.in/wp-content/uploads/2020/05/DPR-All- Press-Notes-dt.-03.05.2020.pdf)

12. Rawat, Mukesh, 'Migrant workers' deaths: Govt says it has no data. But didn't people die? Here is a list', (https://www.indiatoday.in/news-analysis/story/migrant-workers-deaths-govt-says-it-has-no-data-but-didn-t-people-die-here-is-a-list-1722087-2020-09-16)
13. Dutta, Anisha, 'Parliament monsoon session: 97 people died on-board Shramik trains, govt tells Rajya Sabha', (https://www.hindustantimes.com/india-news/parliament-%20monsoon-session-97-people-died-on-board-shramik-trains-govt-%20tells-rajya-sabha/story-AvX2CNUL3QQnQKnkcSC0yM.htm)
14. Centre for Sustainable Employment, Azim Premji University and NREGA Consortium, Faculty Research, 'Employment guarantee during COVID-19: Role of MGNREGA post the 2020 lockdown', (https://azimpremjiuniversity.edu.in/faculty-research/employment-guarantee-during-covid-19-role-of-mgnrega-in-the-year-after-the-2020-lockdown)
15. Centre for Sustainable Employment, Azim Premji University and NREGA Consortium, Faculty Research,'Employment guarantee during COVID-19: Role of MGNREGA post the 2020 lockdown', (https://azimpremjiuniversity.edu.in/faculty-research/employment-guarantee-during-covid-19-role-of-mgnrega-in-the-year-after-the-2020-lockdown)
16. Taskin, Bismee, Yadav, Jyoti, 'UP migrants reach Hardoi from Punjab by train, but are then told to find their own way home', (https://theprint.in/india/up-migrants-reach-hardoi-from-punjab-by-train-but-are-then-told-to-find-their-own-way-home/417851/)
17. G Dastidar, Avishek, '1.06 cr migrants returned from cities to home states during lockdown: Govt', (https://indianexpress.com/article/india/1-06-cr-migrants-returned-from-cities-to-home-states-during-lockdown-govt-6606918/)
18. Sharma, Unnati, 'Over 81,000 road accidents during March-June, but no separate data on migrant deaths, says govt', (https://theprint.in/india/over-81000-road-accidents-during-march-june-but-no-separate-data-on-migrant-deaths-says-govt/508966/)
19. PTI, The Week, 'India's COVID-19 tally crosses 67,000 with highest single-day spike of 4,213', (https://www.theweek.in/news/india/2020/05/11/india-covid19-tally-crosses-67000-highest-single-day-spike-4213.html)

20. Ministry of Home Affairs, Government of India, (https://www.mha.gov.in/sites/default/files/MHA Order Dt. 1.5.2020)
21. Census may be held in 2026 to match delimitation schedule, says Union Minister Kishan Reddy (https://www.thehindu.com/news/national/census-may-be-held-next-year-to-match-delimitation-schedule-says-minister-kishan-reddy/article69522508.ece)
22. Singh, Vijaita, 'Caste census: Hindutva firmly on its side, BJP embraces Oppsition's social justice plank with vigour', (https://economictimes.indiatimes.com/news/politics-and-nation/caste-census-hindutva-firmly-on-its-side-bjp-embraces-oppsitions-social-justice-plank-with-vigour/articleshow/120771869.cms?from=mdr)
23. Kumar, Arun, 'Husband follows wife's footsteps as women change Panchayat politics in Bihar', (https://www.hindustantimes.com/cities/patna-news/husband-%20follows-wife-s-footsteps-as-women-change-panchayat-politics-in-%20bihar-101631782087254.html)
24. Gettleman, Jeffrey, Raj, Suhasini "Lionhearted' Girl Bikes Dad Across India, Inspiring a Nation', (https://www.nytimes.com/2020/05/22/world/asia/india-bicycle-girl-migrants.html)
25. Yadav, Tejashwi, (https://x.com/yadavtejashwi/status/1264533836081147904)
26. PTI, India Today, 'LJP offers to sponsor education of girl who cycled 1,200 km with injured father' (https://www.indiatoday.in/india/story/coronavirus-lockdown-ljp-offers-sponsor-education-girl-cycle-darbhanga-gurgaon-injured-father-1681481-2020-05-24)
27. Tripathi Piyush, Kumar Jha, Binay, 'Health ministry to consider making Darbhanga girl, who cycled for 1200kms, its brand ambassador: Union Minister', (https://timesofindia.indiatimes.com/india/health-ministry-to-consider-making-darbhanga-girl-who-cycled-for-1200kms-its-brand-ambassador-union-minister/articleshow/75923560.cms)
28. India Today Web Desk, 'Super 30 opens door for Jyoti Kumari, the girl who cycled 1200 km with injured father', (https://www.indiatoday.in/education-today/news/story/super-30-opens-door-for-jyoti-kumar-the-girl-who-cycled-1200-km-with-injured-father-1681799-2020-05-25)
29. India Today Web Des, 'If there is potential, Jyoti Kumari will be selected as trainee at National Cycling Academy: Kiren Rijiju', (https://www.indiatoday.in/sports/other-sports/story/kiren-rijiju-

says-jyoti-kumari-to-be-selected-as-trainee-at-national-cycling-academy-if-clears-trials-1681362-2020-05-24)

30. Navbharat times, 'दरभंगा की 'साइकलि गर्ल' ज्योतकि को राष्ट्रीय बाल पुरस्कार, पीएम मोदी ने दयिा सफलता का मंत्र', (https://navbharattimes.indiatimes.com/state/bihar/darbhanga/pm-narendra-modi-interacts-rashtriya-bal-puraskar-awardees-darbhanga-girl-jyoti-kumari-honored-pmrbp-video-conference/articleshow/80445751.cms)

2. 2021. THE DANCE OF DEATH IN LUCKNOW

1. PTI, NDTV, 'UP Records Highest-Ever Single Day Spike Of 15,353 New COVID-19 Cases', (https://www.ndtv.com/india-news/up-records-highest-ever-single-day-spike-of-15-353-new-covid-19-cases-2411367)
2. India News, 'People are now dying on roads', Lucknow DM video goes viral', (https://www.indiatvnews.com/video/news/people-are-now-dying-%20on-roads-lucknow-dm-video-goes-viral-697698)
3. PTI, NDTV, 'Uttar Pradesh Records Highest-Ever Daily Spike Of 18,021 COVID-19 Cases', (https://www.ndtv.com/india-news/uttar-pradesh-records-highest-ever-daily-spike-of-18-021-covid-19-cases-2412976)
4. Rashid, Omar, 'Coronavirus | U.P. to shut schools, coaching centres till April 30', (https://www.thehindu.com/news/national/other-states/coronavirus-up-to-shut-schools-coaching-centres-till-april-30/article34295708.ece)
5. Night curfew hours extended in 10 UP cities (https://www.etvbharat.com/english/state/uttar-pradesh/night-curfew-hours-extended-in-10-up-cities/na20210415172256654)
6. Yadav, Jyoti, "Dead bodies all over': Lucknow funerals tell a story starkly different from UP govt's claims', (https://theprint.in/india/dead-bodies-all-over-lucknow-funerals-tell-a-story-starkly-different-from-up-govts-claims/640741/)
7. Sharda, Shailvee, 'UP: Death toll crosses 100; 22,439 new Covid cases in 24 hours', (https://timesofindia.indiatimes.com/city/lucknow/death-toll-crosses-100-22439-new-covid-cases-in-24-hours/articleshow/82092889.cms)
8. Yadav, Jyoti,'Dead bodies all over': Lucknow funerals tell a story starkly different from UP govt's claims', (https://theprint.in/india/dead-bodies-all-over-lucknow-funerals-tell-a-story-starkly-different-from-up-govts-claims/640741/)

3. A DEATH LIVE-TWEETED

1. Kumar, Ravi Prakash, 'Coronavirus treatment: Ramdev's Patanjali launches Coronil kit for ₹545', (https://www.livemint.com/news/india/coronavirusvaccine-coronil-patanjali-baba-ramdev-press conference-live-updates-11592893304534.html)
2. Sharma, Sanjay, 'Patanjali sold 25 lakh Coronil kits worth Rs 250 crore in 4 months', (https://www.indiatoday.in/india/story/patanjali sold-25-lakh-coronil-kits-worth-rs-250-crore-in-4-months-1737229-2020-11-02)
3. Sharma, Milan, 'Ayush ministry allows sale of Patanjali's Coronil as immunity booster', (https://www.indiatoday.in/india/story/ayush-ministry allows-sale-of-patanjali-s-coronil-as-immunity booster-1695911-2020-07-01)
4. The Week, 'Baba Ramdev's Patanjali says Coronil is the first evidence-based medicine to fight COVID-19', (https://www.theweek.in/news/india/2021/02/19/ baba-ramdev-patanjali-says-coronil-is-the-first evidence-based-medicine-to-fight-covid-19.html)
5. ANI, 'Baba Ramdev launches Patanjali's 'evidence based' medicine for Covid-19' (https://economictimes.indiatimes.com/industry/healthcare/biotech/pharmaceuticals/baba-ramdev launches-patanjalis-evidence-based-medicine-for covid-19/videoshow/81106154.cms)
6. Special Correspondent, 'IMA 'shocked' over Patanjali's claim on Coronil; demands explanation from Harsh Vardhan', (https://www.thehindu.com/news/national/imashocked-over-patanjalis-claim-on-coronil-demandsexplanation-from-harsh-vardhan/article 33902720.ece)
7. HT News Desk, 'Wilful disobedience': Supreme Court slams Baba Ramdev, Acharya Balkrishna, rejects apology', (https://www.hindustantimes.com/india-news/wilfuldisobedience-supreme-court-slams-baba-ramdevacharya-balkrishna-rejects apology-101712732394427.html)
8. Mukherjee, Vasudha, 'SC closes contempt case as Ramdev, Balkrishna agree to end misleading ads', (https://www.business-standard.com/india-news/sccloses-contempt-case-as-ramdev-balkrishna-agree to-end-misleading-ads-124081300555_1.html)
9. Yadav, Jyoti, 'Where are ambulances, Covid hospitals?': Family of UP journalist who died without treatment', (https://theprint.

in/health/where-are-ambulances covid-hospitals-family-of-up-journalist-who-died without-treatment/641750/)

10. Times of India, PM Modi's interview with ANI: Full transcript',(https://timesofindia.indiatimes.com/india/pm-modis interview-with-ani-full-transcript/articleshow/ 109322017.cms)
11. Modi ki Gurantee, Bhartiya Janta Party, 'BJP's Manifesto General Election 2024 | BJP Sankalp Patra 2024', (https://www.bjp.org/pressreleases/bjps-manifestogeneral-election-2024-bjp-sankalp-patra-2024)

4. OVERBURDENED SMALLER TOWNS

1. Staff report, The New Indian Express, 'UP's COVID death toll surpasses 10,000 mark; state faces oxygen, beds' shortage', (https://www.newindianexpress.com/nation/2021/ Apr/21/ups-covid-death-toll-surpasses-10000-mark state-faces-oxygen-beds-shortage-2292779.html)
2. Ahsan, Sofi, 'Delhi High Court to Centre: Beg, borrow, steal, it's your job to get oxygen', (https://indianexpress.com/article/cities/delhi/delhihigh-court-centre-oxygen-supply-hospitals covid-19-7283552/)

5. A BREATHLESS CITY

1. Srivastava, Prashant, 'In new UP system for Covid hospital admission, doctors will take call, not CMO', (https://theprint.in/india/governance/in-new-up system-for-covid-hospital-admission-doctors-will take-call-not-cmo/643563/)
2. Srivastava, Samarth, 'Death of Covid patients due to non-supply of oxygen not less than genocide: Allahabad HC' (https://www.indiatoday.in/coronavirus-outbreak/story/covid-patients-death-non-supply-of-oxygengenocide-allahabad-high court-1798953-2021-05-05)
3. Rashid, Omar , 'Oxygen shortage | Seize property of those spreading rumours: Yogi Adityanath', (https://www.thehindu.com/news/national/other states/seize-property-of-those-spreading-rumours up-cm/article34404518.ece)
4. Moole, Janhavee, 'A nightmare on repeat - India is running out of oxygen again', (https://www.bbc.com/news/uk-56841381)
5. Prime Minister's Office, Government of India, 'PM CARES Fund Trust allocates Rs 201.58 crores for installation of 162 dedicated

PSA Medical Oxygen Generation Plants in public health facilities', (https://www.pib.gov.in/Pressreleaseshare.aspx? PRID=1686271)

6. Rajya Sabha, Unstarred question number 920, Ministry of Health and Family Welfare, 'PRESSURE SWING ADSORPTION OXYGEN PLANTS', (https://sansad.in/getFile/annex/254/AU920.pdf? source=pqars)
7. Ministry of Health and Family Welfare (MoHFW), (https://x.com/MoHFW_INDIA/status/ 1383651682270072846)
8. PTI, NDTV, 'Nearly 8,700 Tonnes Of Liquid Medical Oxygen Delivered Across India: Railways', (https://www.ndtv.com/india-news/oxygen-express railways-says-it-has-delivered-nearly-8-700-tonnes of-liquid-medical-oxygen-across-india-2442456)
9. Staff writer, Mint, 'Indian Air Force flown 1,400 hours in 21 days to boost oxygen supply', (https://www.livemint.com/news/india/indian-air force-flown-1-400-hours-in-21-days-to-boost oxygen-supply-11620815947801.html)
10. PTI, Economic times, 'COVID-19: Tender to be floated to import 50,000 MT of medical oxygen, says Centre', (https://economictimes.indiatimes.com/news/india/covid-19-tender-to-be-floated-to-import-50000-mt-of-medical-oxygen-says-centre/articleshow/82089420.cms)
11. Perappadan, Bindu Shajan, 'Parliament proceedings | No deaths reported due to lack of oxygen, Health Ministry tells Rajya Sabha', (https://www.thehindu.com/news/national/parliament proceedings-no-deaths-reported-due-to-lack-ofoxygen-health-ministry-tells-rajya-sabha/ article35428791.ece)
12. Scroll Staff, 'No Covid-19 deaths reported in Uttar Pradesh due to oxygen shortage, claims state health minister', (https://scroll.in/latest/1012983/no-covid-19-deaths reported-%20in-uttar-pradesh-due-to-oxygen shortage-claims-state-health-%20minister)
13. Office of the Registrar General & Census Commissioner, India (ORGI), 'REPORT ON VITAL STATISTICS OF INDIA BASED ON THE CIVIL REGISTRATION SYSTEM-2021', (https://censusindia.gov.in/nada/index.php/catalog/ 45554)

7. DYING LIKE FLIES: A TALE OF TWO VARANASI VILLAGES

1. Special Correspondent, 'Coronavirus | India becomes first country in the world to report over 4 lakh new cases in a single day on April 30, 2021', (https://www.thehindu.com/news/national/ coronavirus-

india- becomes-first-country-in-the world-to-report-over-400000-new- cases-on april-30-2021/article61817889.ece)

2. Yadav, Jyoti, 'The young in these 2 Varanasi villages started to die. That's when Covid became 'real', (https://theprint.in/india/the-young-in-these-2-varanasi-villages-started-to-die-thats-when-covid became-real/646326/)

8. THE RETURNED MIGRANTS IN JAUNPUR

1. PTI, NDTV, UP Panchayat Polls To Be Held In 4 Phases Starting April 15', (https://www.ndtv.com/india-news/up-panchayatelection-date-2021-uttar-pradesh-panchayat-pollsphases-starting-date-april-15-2399646)

2. Kumar, Anshuman, Ex IAS officer and BJP MLC AK Sharma steps in to control worsening Varanasi pandemic', (https://economictimes.indiatimes.com/news/india/ak-sharma-steps-in-to-control-worsening-varanasipandemic/articleshow/82072350.cms?from=mdr)

10. THE DEADLY PANCHAYAT POLLS

1. Supreme Court of India, Ram Sharan Maurya vs State Of U. P. on 18 November, 2020', (https://indiankanoon.org/doc/47374276/)

2. Mishra, Abhishek, UP govt releases compensation for kin of over 2,000 employees who died of Covid during panchayat polls', (https://www.indiatoday.in/india/story/up-govtreleases-compensation-kin-over-2000-employeessuccumbed-to-covid-panchayat polls-1849003-2021-09-03)

3. Hindustan Times Correspondent, '700 govt school staff died on poll duty: UP teachers' body writes to CM, EC', (https://www.hindustantimes.com/india-news/700- govt- school-staff-died-on-poll-duty-up-teachers body-writes-to-cm- ec-101619812988669.html)

4. Rashid, Omar, 'U.P. panchayat elections turned deadly for those on duty', (https://www.thehindu.com/news/national/other states/ up-panchayat-elections-turned-deadly-forthose-on-duty/ article34442370.ece)

5. Hindustan Times Correspondent, '700 govt school staff died on poll duty: UP teachers' body writes to CM, EC', (https://www.hindustantimes.com/india-news/700-govt-school-staff-died-on-poll-duty-up-teachersbody-writes-to-cm-ec-101619808408780.html)

6. Mishra, Abhishek, Unions say 577 teachers died on Uttar Pradesh panchayat poll duty,' (https://www.indiatoday.in/india/story/uttar-pradeshteachers-unions-577-teachers-died-panchayat-pollduty-1796282-2021-04-29)
7. IANS, Buisness Standard, Allahabad HC issues notice to UPSEC over death of 135 teachers on poll duty,' (https://www.business-standard.com/article/current affairs/allahabad-hc-issues-notice-to-upsec-overdeath-of-135-teachers-on-pollduty-121042800115_1.html)
8. Netional Herald Correspondent, 'Yogi government blames High Court for Panchayat polls,' (https://www.nationalheraldindia.com/india/yogi government-blames-high-court-for-panchayat-polls)
9. Hindustan Times Correspondent, 'Over 700 staff on poll duty in UP lostbattleto Covid-19': Teachers' body,' (https://www.hindustantimes.com/cities/lucknownews/over-700-staff-on-poll-duty-in-up-lost-battleto-covid-19-teachers-body-101619788548468.html)
10. Rashid, Omar, U.P. teachers unions call off boycott of panchayat polls counting,' (https://www.thehindu.com/news/national/other states/up-teachers-unions-call-off-boycott-ofpanchayat-polls-counting/article34460195.ece)
11. Gaur, Vatsala, 'Only 3 teachers died on panchayat poll duty; to be given compensation: UP government,' (https://economictimes.indiatimes.com/news/politics-and-nation/only-3-teachers-died-on panchayat-poll-duty-to-be-given-compensation-upgovernment/articleshow/82762170. cms?from=mdr)
12. Mullick, Rajeev, 'Not 1,609, 3 teachers died on poll duty: UP govt', (https://www.hindustantimes.com/india-news/not-1-609-3-teachers-died-on-poll-duty up-101621363634623.html)
13. Shrivastava, Samarth , 'UP govt to give Rs 30 lakh aid to kin of panchayat polls workers who died of Covid-19', (https://www.indiatoday.in/india/story/up-govt-rs-30- lakh-aid-to- panchayat-polls-workers families-1809316-2021-06-01)
14. Jain, Ritika, 'Pay ₹1 Cr Damages To Polling Officers Who Died Of COVID: Allahabad HC', (https://www.boomlive.in/law/allahabad-high-court uttar- pradesh-panchayat-elections-135- dead-13127)
15. Mishra, Abhishek, 'UP govt releases compensation for kin of over 2,000 employees who died of Covid during panchayat polls', (https://www.indiatoday.in/india/story/up-govtreleases-

compensation-kin-over-2000-employeessuccumbed-to-covid-panchayat polls-1849003-2021-09-03)
16. Srivastava, Adarsh, 'Supreme Court upholds BTC eligibility for primary teachers, BEd excluded from Level-1 teaching jobs', (https://www.indiatvnews.com/jobs/news/supreme court-upholds-btc-eligibility-for-primary-teachersbed-excluded-from-level-1-teaching jobs-2023-08-12-886236)

11. BUXAR: A DISTRICT WITHOUT A FUNCTIONAL VENTILATOR

1. Ministry of Health and Family Welfare, 'Government of India announces a Liberalised and Accelerated Phase 3 Strategy of Covid-19 Vaccination from 1st May', (https://www.pib.gov.in/PressReleasePage.aspx? PRID=1712710)
2. Ministry of Health and Family Welfare, 'Government of India announces a Liberalised and Accelerated Phase 3 Strategy of Covid-19 Vaccination from 1st May', (https://www.pib.gov.in/PressReleasePage.aspx? PRID=1712710)
3. PTI, 'Serum Institute of India restarts manufacturing of COVID-19 vaccine Covishield', (https://indianexpress.com/article/india/serum institute-of-india-restarts-manufacturing-covid-19-vaccine-covishield-8552970/)
4. Kaul, Rhythma, 'Elderly, those with chronic diseases to get vaccine first: Harsh Vardhan', (https://www.hindustantimes.com/india-news/elderly-those-with-chronic-diseases-to-get-vaccinefirst-harsh-vardhan/story mtvgBVpOQQHeDgz8GKsDQP.html)
5. Koshy, Jacob , 'Vaccines for all above 18 from May 1; States can buy directly', (https://www.thehindu.com/news/national/frommay-1-everyone-over-18-years-eligible-for-covid-19-vaccination-government/ article34359940.ece)
6. Koshy, Jacob , 'Vaccines for all above 18 from May 1; States can buy directly', (https://www.thehindu.com/news/national/frommay-1-everyone-over-18-years-eligible-for-covid-19-vaccination-government/ article34359940.ece)
7. NDTV News Desk, "Don't Queue Up For Vaccines Tomorrow": Arvind Kejriwal Amid Shortage', (https://www.ndtv.com/india-news/coronavirusarvind-kejriwal-tells-delhi-residents-dont-queue-upfor-vaccines-tomorrow-says-people-will-beinformed-once-stocks-are-in-2425108)

8. PTI, Business Standard, 'Over 86,000 people in 18-44 years age group receive first dose on May 1', (https://www.business-standard.com/article/current affairs/over- 86-000-people-in-18-44-years-age group-receive-first-dose-on-may-1-121050200296_1.html)
9. Scroll Staff, 'Coronavirus: Bihar imposes lockdown till May 15 after Patna HC pulls up government for case surge', (https://scroll.in/latest/994024/coronavirus-biharimposes-lockdown-till-may-15-after-patna-hc-pulls up-government-for-case-surge)
10. Yadav, Jyoti, 'Surprise, surprise, Bihar's Buxar has 6 ventilators. No surprise: No one to operate them', (https://theprint.in/india/bihars-buxar-is-fighting covid-surge-with- ventilators-that-dont-work-or-are locked-up/65186)

12. 'JO HOSPITAL JAYEGA WOH MAARA JAYEGA'

1. PTI, India TV, 'Bihar: PMCH to get Rs 5540 cr 'world class' makeover', (https://www.indiatvnews.com/news/india/pmch patna-makeover-project-rs-5540-cr-nitish-kumar lays-foundation-stone-details-683564)
2. 'Yadav, Jyoti, 'Jo hospital jayega woh maara jayega': Why no one wants to go to Patna's top govt facilities', (https://theprint.in/health/better-to-die-at-home-why covid-patients-have-lost-faith-in-two-of-patnas-govt hospitals/655299/)

13. QUACKS IN RURAL BIHAR

1. Sharma, Neetu Chandra m 'Why do quacks function freely in India?', (https://www.livemint.com/Science/BFelCnQ2fp120Kf5dhBQZP/Why-do-quacks function-freely-in-India.html)
2. Ali, Sajid, Bihar's Bhojpur, quacks are 'Gods who save lives' as hospitals battle Covid burden', (https://theprint.in/health/in-bihars-bhojpur-quacks-are-gods- who-save-lives-as-hospitals-battle-covid burden/655674/)
3. Chandna, Himani, Just 1 doctor to treat 11,000 patients: The scary truth of India's govt healthcare', (https://theprint.in/india/governance/just-1-doctor-totreat-11000-patients-govt-report-details-indias health-crisis/74013/)
4. Yadav, Jyoti, In Arrah & Buxar, pharmacists and 'jhola chaaps' are treating Covid because doctors 'refuse to', (https://theprint.in/health/in-arrah-buxar-pharmacists and-jhola-chaaps-are-treating-covid-because doctors-refuse-to/657221/)

14. THE COVID ORPHANS

1. Tripathi, Piyush, Kamlesh K, 'Bihar govt blames Uttar Pradesh for bodies washing ashore in Buxar', (https://timesofindia.indiatimes.com/city/patna/bihar govt-blames-uttar-pradesh-for-bodies-washing ashore-in-buxar/articleshow/82556643.cms)
2. Yadav, Jyoti, Covid killed parents, 3 Bihar siblings now fight virus stigma — 'no one even offered food', (https://theprint.in/india/covid-killed-parents-3-bihar siblings-now-fight-virus-stigma-no-one-even offered-food/657771/)
3. Kumar, Madan, Bihar govt paying Rs 4 lakh ex-gratia to next kin of Covid victimes from the CM relief fund: Nitish Kumar', (https://timesofindia.indiatimes.com/city/patna/bihar govt-paying-rs-4-lakh-ex-gratia-to-next-kin-of covid-victimes-from-the-cm-relief-fund-nitish-kumar/ articleshow/82918930.cms)
4. Ministry of Women and Child Development, Government of India, 'Lancet Article Sophisticated Trickery Intended To Create Panic Among Citizens, Divorced From Truth And Ground Reality: Ministry Of Women And Child Development', (https://www.pib.gov.in/PressReleaseIframePage.aspx?PRID=1802393)
5. The Lancet Child & Adolescent Health, 'Global, regional, and national minimum estimates of children affected by COVID-19-associated orphanhood and caregiver death, by age and family circumstance up to Oct 31, 2021: an updated modelling study', (https://www.thelancet.com/journals/lanchi/article/PIIS2352-4642(22)00005-0/fulltext)
6. Hindustan Times Correspondent, 'Sophisticated trickery': Govt rebuts Lancet study on children affected by pandemic', (https://www.hindustantimes.com/india-news/sophisticated-trickery-govt-rebuts-lancet-study-on children-affected-by-pandemic-101646251865370.html)
7. PTI, The HIndu, 'Over half of PM CARES for Children scheme applications for COVID orphans rejected', (https://www.thehindu.com/news/national/over-half of-pm-cares-for-children-scheme-applications-for covid-orphans-rejected/ article68409285.ece)
8. Yadav, Jyoti, 'Red-eyed, lost young men in Bihar's Seemanchal show how Nitish Kumar's alcohol ban backfired', (https://theprint.in/feature/red-eyed-lost-young-men in-bihars-seemanchal-show-how-nitish-kumars alcohol-ban- backfired/891957/)
9. Santhya, K.G. Acharya, Rajib Pandey, Neelanjana Kumar Singh,

Santosh Rampal, Shilpi Francis Zavier, A.J. Kumar Gupta, Ashish, 'Understanding the lives of adolescents and young adults (UDAYA) in Bihar, India', (https://www.projectudaya.in/wp-content/uploads/2018/08/Bihar-Report-pdf.pdf)

10. Jeffrey, Craig ,'Generation Nowhere': rethinking youth through the lens of unemployed young men', (https://journals.sagepub.com/doi/10.1177/0309132507088119)

15. IF THERE IS A HELL, IT IS HERE

1. (https://theprint.in/health/if-theres-hell-its-here-a-day-with-patients-in-dmch-north-bihars-mainstay-hospital/661173/)

16. THE LAST LEG

1. The Ministry of Health and Family Welfare, 'COVID-19 Statewise Status', (https://covid19dashboard.mohfw.gov.in/)
2. World Health Organisation, 'Weekly epidemiological update on COVID-19 - 25 May 2021', (https://www.who.int/publications/m/item/weekly epidemiological-update-on-covid-19---25-may-2021)
3. Economic Times, 'Patwa toli: The village of IITians in Bihar', (https://economictimes.indiatimes.com/news/india/ patwa-toli-the- village-of-iitians-in-bihar/articleshow/ 109139545.cms?from=mdr)
4. Yadav, Jyoti, 'This Bihar weaver's business is booming as demand for kafans rise, and he's not a happy man', (https://theprint.in/india/this-bihar-weavers-business is-booming- but-hes-not-a-happy-man/667544/)
5. Yadav, Jyoti, 'Bihar family hides mom's Covid infection from villagers, but feeds 600 at her funeral feast', (https://theprint.in/india/bihar-family-hides-moms covid- infec tion-f rom-villagers-but-feeds-600-at-her funeral- feast/669739/)
6. Yadav, Jyoti, 'We travel 22km to send a WhatsApp' — vaccine slot a distant reality for 118 Bihar villages (https://theprint.in/health/we-travel-22km-to-send-a whatsapp-vaccine-slot-a-distant-reality-for-118- bihar-villages/671187/)
7. A female health worker based at a health sub centre or primary health centre. They are the essential frontline workers under the National Rural Health Mission.
8. Sheriff M, Kaunain, 'India's journey towards 100-crore vaccine milestone in just over 9 months' (https://indianexpress.com/

article/india/india-100-crore-covid-19-vaccine-milestone-timeline-7582970/)

9. Press Information Bureau, Government of India, 'NATIONAL COVID-19 VACCINATION',(https://www.pib.gov.in/PressReleseDetailm.aspx? PRID=1894907).
10. Press Information Bureau, Government of India, 'India's Pharma Exports grow over 125% in last 9 years Investment of Rs. 21,861 Crore received under PLI Schemes', (https://www.pib.gov.in/PressReleasePage.aspx?PRID=1931918#:%20~:text=Further,%20India%20has%20supplied%20over,till%20May %2019,%202023)

Acknowledgements

My deepest gratitude to—

my grandfather and grandmother, Ramchandra and Sarti Devi, who devoted their entire pension towards my education in Delhi, enabling me to become the first person in the family to earn a postgraduate degree, and the first girl to travel and live beyond the realms of our house and fields;

my mother, Saroj, who took it upon herself to wage a war on my behalf whenever someone in the family or neighbourhood stood against the idea of educating a girl, or letting her buy a laptop, or allowing her to board the Haryana roadways transport that would take her to Delhi. She gave me agency;

my Bua-ji, for her kindness. She would slip me pocket money on many occasions for those bus rides;

my school teachers, Praveen Sir, Dinesh Sir, and Satyapal master from Sarvodya School, who planted the idea in my elder brother Naveen's mind that a student like me deserved to go to a bigger university, rather than a JBT course in the nearby town, the most freedom granted to the girls around me;

Naveen bhai, who made several train journeys from Gudha railway station to Delhi's stations, until he finally helped me secure admission into Daulat Ram College;

Delhi University—for opening up a world of possibilities for me, for helping me find my voice;

my professors, my batchmates and friends, who made space for the person I became in the subsequent years;

Dilli, the city where I first arrived as a sixteen-year-old girl. It is where I spent my twenties, exploring, making mistakes, learning, and unlearning. The city remains an overarching figure in my life. People often attribute toxic masculine traits to it, but to me, Dilli is like an old tiger mom, who gave me autonomy and the audacity to be myself;

the English Literature course, which was a turning point for me, where I read Shakespeare, Virginia Woolf, and Simone de Beauvoir, through the lens of my raw Haryanvi sensibilities;

my first job at the India Today Group, which was foundational in my career.

This book was born of an unspoken social contract between a journalist and the public. It was born of a connection that allows journalists to step into people's lives and witness events that may be very personal to them, especially death.

The interviews that formed the corpus I drew on while writing this book were not conducted in ordinary times. Migrants—men, women and little children—paused mid-journey to speak to me. Some stepped down from the trucks they were travelling on; many rested their weary feet after walking hundreds of kilometres with their entire lives bundled on their backs. Some people spoke to me while bidding goodbye to their loved ones at cremation grounds; others talked as they sat beside the corpses of family members in hospital wards. Their grief was raw, and when they ran out of words, they spoke through tears. I have tried to stitch together their words, tears and ordeals in this book.

You won't find all the people I met during my assignment within its pages, but I want to take this opportunity to thank every single one of them for the kindness they bestowed upon me by opening their doors and handing me gamchchas and tiffin boxes as I trudged through UP and Bihar in the relentless April and May heat.

The drivers I travelled with are the backbone of my coverage of COVID. The company of Arunesh, Babloo, Manish, Chhotu and Binod kept me safe and sane.

I am grateful to—my colleague Bismee Taskin, with whom I had the privilege of sharing the Ramnath Goenka Award for our coverage of the migrant exodus; Shekhar Gupta, editor-in-chief at *ThePrint*. I became a reporter because of his conviction. When I first met him in 2019, I barely knew the ABCs of ground reporting. Thank you, Shekhar, for giving Hindiwallahs the chance they deserved. Thank you for bringing me out of the corner Hindi desk to the English one. You have no idea how much confidence it instilled in me every time you turned to me at the beginning of editorial meetings—'Haan Jyoti, batao kya news hai?'; Rama Lakshmi, my dream editor, whom I closely observed in meetings. Her sharp gaze and articulation left a lasting impression on me. Every time I walked past her cabin, all I wanted to say was, 'Take me in your team.' She is the one who gave the book its title, *Faith and Fury*. Between her and Shekhar, I truly feel I lucked out; my Hindi editor, the late Renu Agal, who left us in 2021; Y.P. Rajesh, who led the coverage through both waves, D.K. Singh, political editor, and Jyoti Malhotra, who headed the video team at the time; Pooja Mehrotra, Tarun Krishna, Gaurav Singh, Inder Belag, Rahul Sampal and Prashant Srivastava, with whom I worked in the Hindi team; my colleagues whose work bolstered me as they reported from different states: Simrin Sirur, Aneesha Bedi, Fatima Khan, Unnati Sharma, Shubhangi Misra, Urjita Bhardwaj, Ananya Bhardwaj, Soniya Agrawal and Moushumi Das Gupta; the rockstars at the desk, who juggled late-night shifts and edited the stories with sensitivity and urgency: Sanghamitra Majumdar, Sunanda Ranjan, Poulomi Banerjee, Shreyas Sharma, Myithili Hazarika, Neera Majumdar, Prashant Dixit, Priyanjali Mitra; Upendra Yadav, Sajid Ali, Vindhesh and Sunil; Suraj Singh Bisht, Manisha Mondal and Praveen Jain from the photography team; Soham Sen, who made powerful graphics for the stories; and the womanhood at *ThePrint*—it is a rare Indian newsroom, where women outnumber men.

I am also thankful to Minakshi Thakur, my editor and publisher at Westland Books, for her rare patience and commitment. Over the last five years, books have come and gone, but she never lost sight of this one. I am grateful to the administrators, ASHA workers, doctors, nurses and frontline workers who shared insights and data, providing context to my ground reports, even if many of them wished to remain anonymous. I can't thank enough the readers, who breathe oxygen into long-form journalism in the age of thirty-second reels.

Thank you, Vandana Menon, for reading the prologue to this manuscript and giving valuable advice; Unnati Sharma, for reading the many drafts and not letting me abandon this book; my dearest friend Tabeenah Anjum, also for reading the drafts diligently; and Harshita Sachan, my best friend, as well as Kanika, for helping me arrive at its final shape.

My heartfelt thanks to my parents-in-law, Sambhu Prasad and Ragini, and my sister-in-law, Nitu, for the love and warmth they have given to me. And lastly, to Rahul, my partner, my home, my cheerleader, always standing like a rock behind me, letting me shine, stepping back when needed, and celebrating me. Everyone talks about empowering women, but not everyone makes space for the empowered woman. Thank you for making that space for me, and our daughter Imara. None of this would have been possible without you.

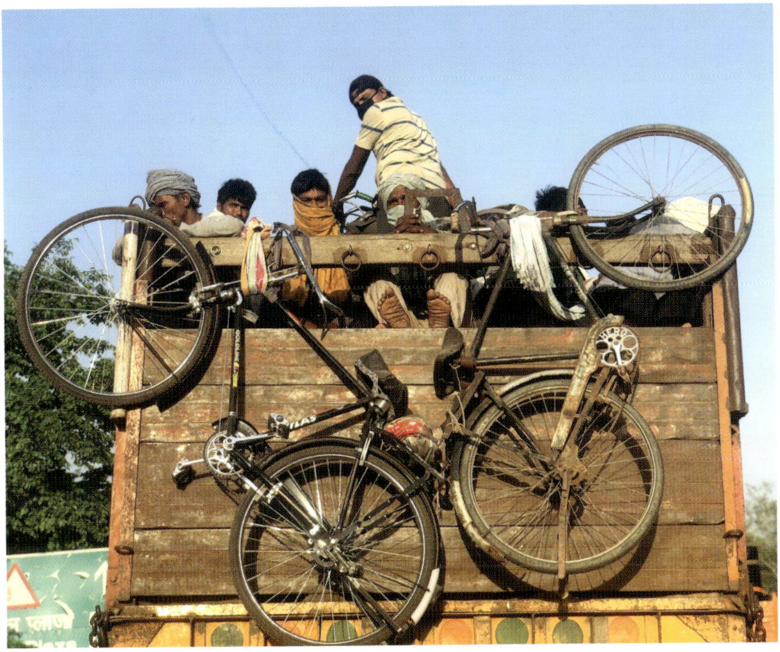

A group of migrants on its journey home

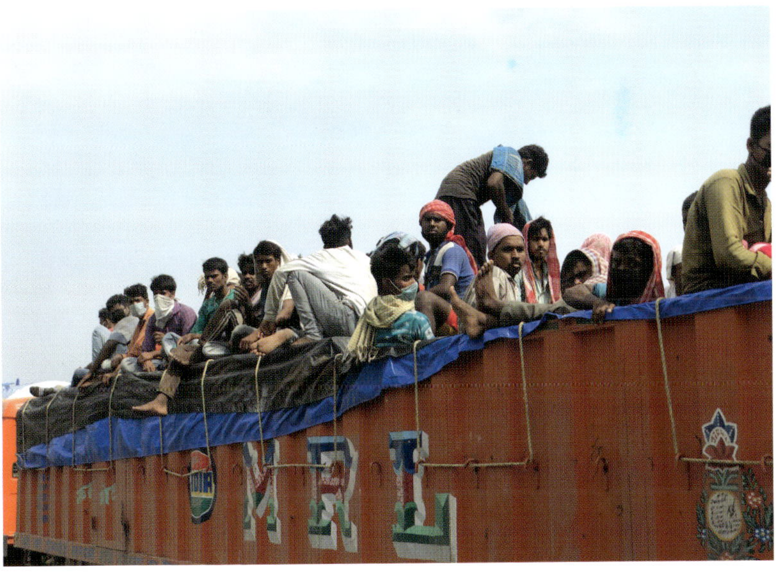

Faces covered with handkerchiefs or gamchhas, migrants sat huddled atop trucks often loaded with iron rods, stones and other cargo, in the scorching heat of May.

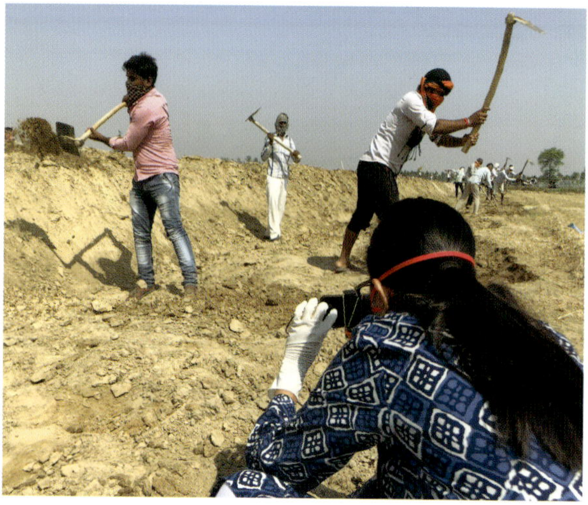

Bilpur in Faridpur Tehsil, located at the border of Shahjahanpur and Bareilly districts, where returned migrants during the nationwide lockdown were engaged in MGNREGA work at a daily wage of 202 rupees

A government school in Sitamarhi district, Bihar, was converted into a quarantine centre for migrants returning to their villages. Mosquito nets were distributed by the state. Classroom benches were used as makeshift beds.

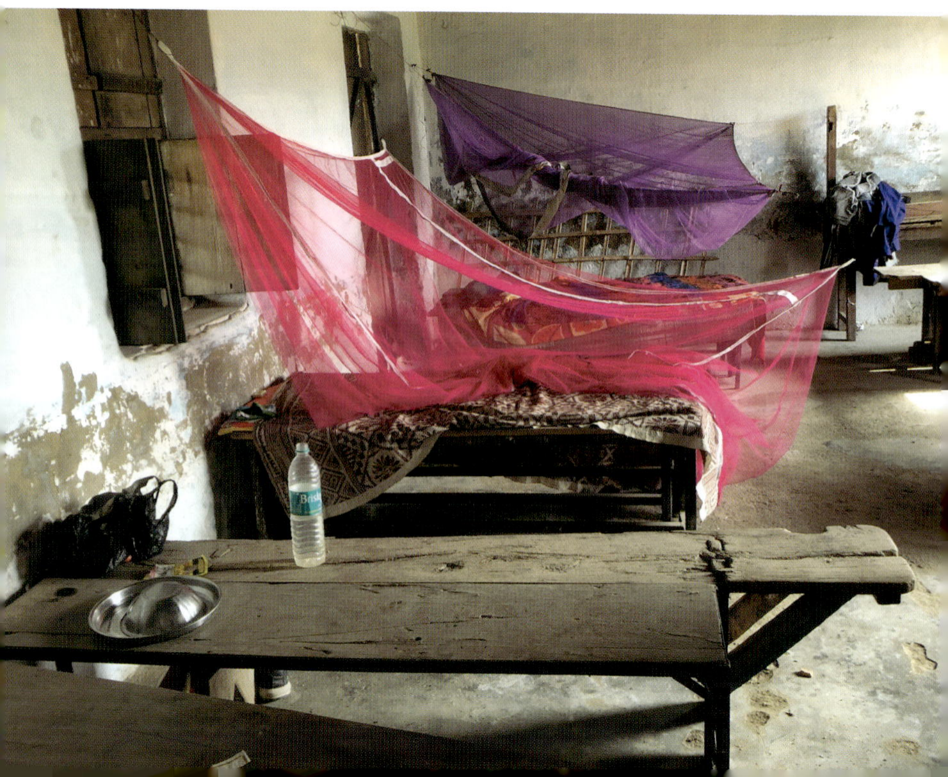

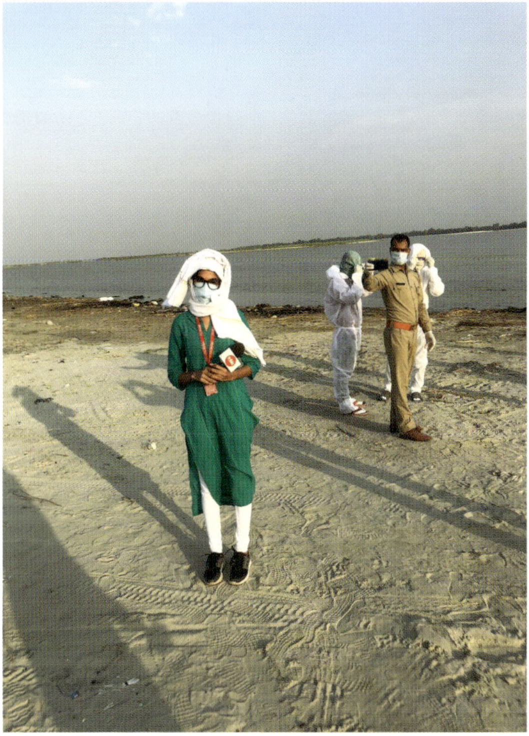

The last rites of migrant Ram Kripal from Haiser village in Sant Kabir Nagar. I was preparing for a piece to camera for a video story before the funeral began. Behind me, a policeman was taking a selfie while the Doms, the cremators, readied themselves to perform the rites.

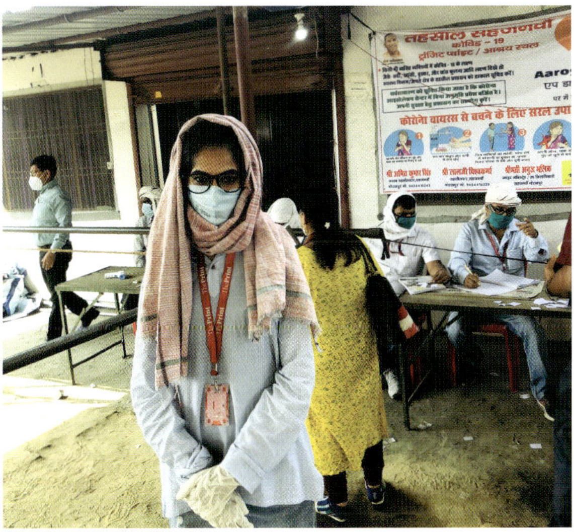

13 May 2020. At a screening centre near the Gorakhpur–Gopalganj border.

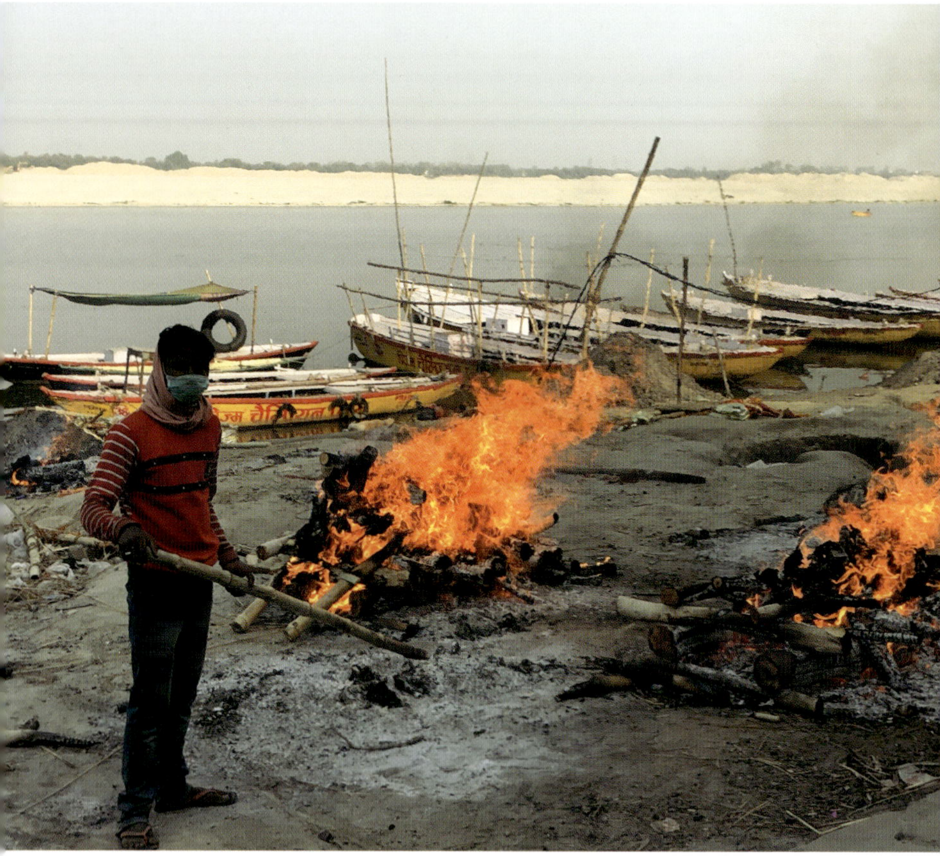

Varanasi, 29 April 2021. At Manikarnika Ghat,
a Dom (cremator) tends to multiple pyres simultaneously.

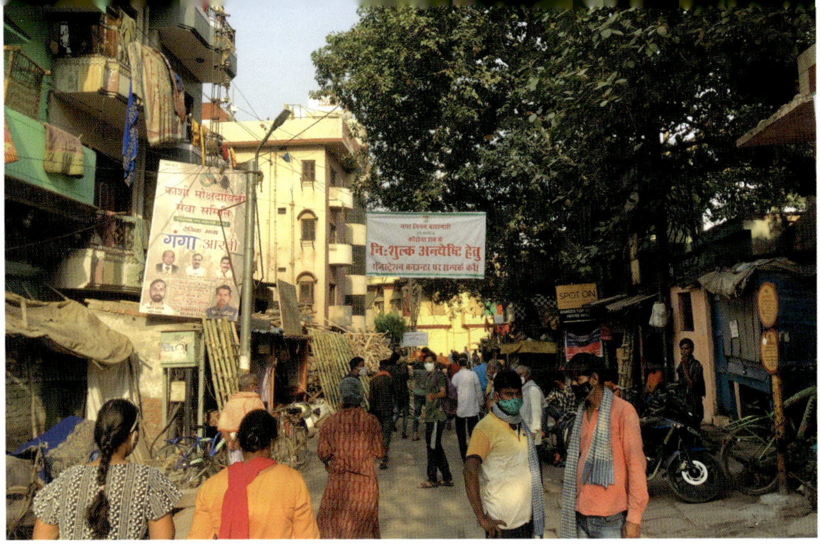

A banner by the Municipal Corporation of Varanasi announced that it would cremate the bodies of COVID-19 victims free of cost. Due to fear and stigma, many COVID-positive bodies were abandoned, denying them the dignity of a funeral by loved ones. The Doms (cremators) took it upon themselves to pick up these bodies from various hospital wards and houses, and perform their last rites.

Varanasi, 29 April 2021. A group of Doms (cremators) taking a short break at Manikarnika Ghat. Most worked without protective gear, tending to the dead day and night.

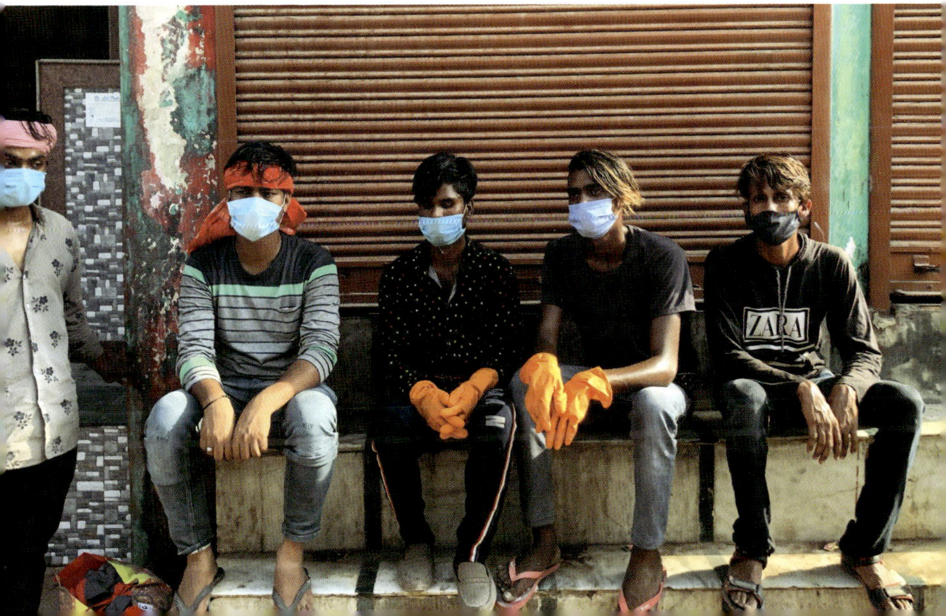

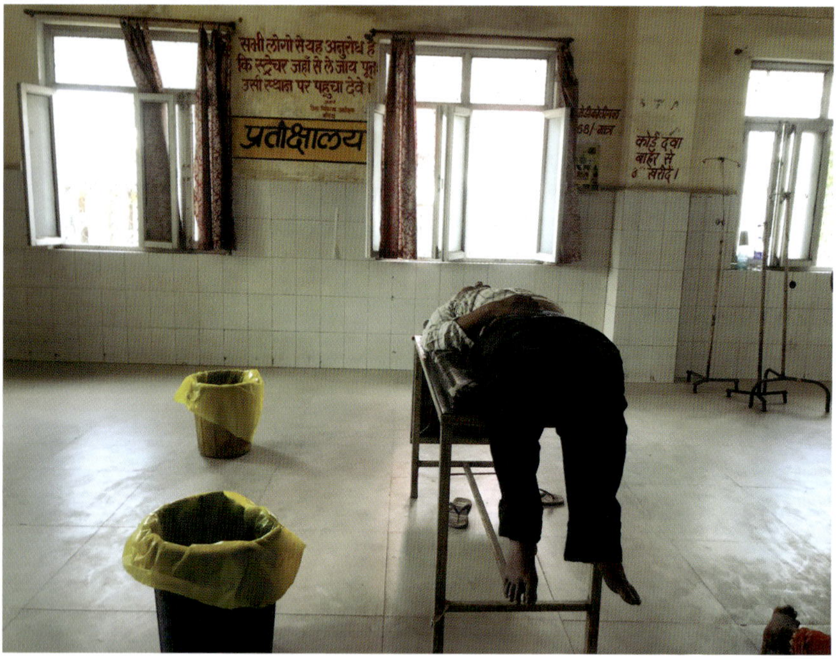

In the general ward of Ballia District Hospital, Uttar Pradesh, the dead body of a man lay among the living on 27 April 2021. Who he was, where he came from and who he belonged to—there was no trace of the man's family.

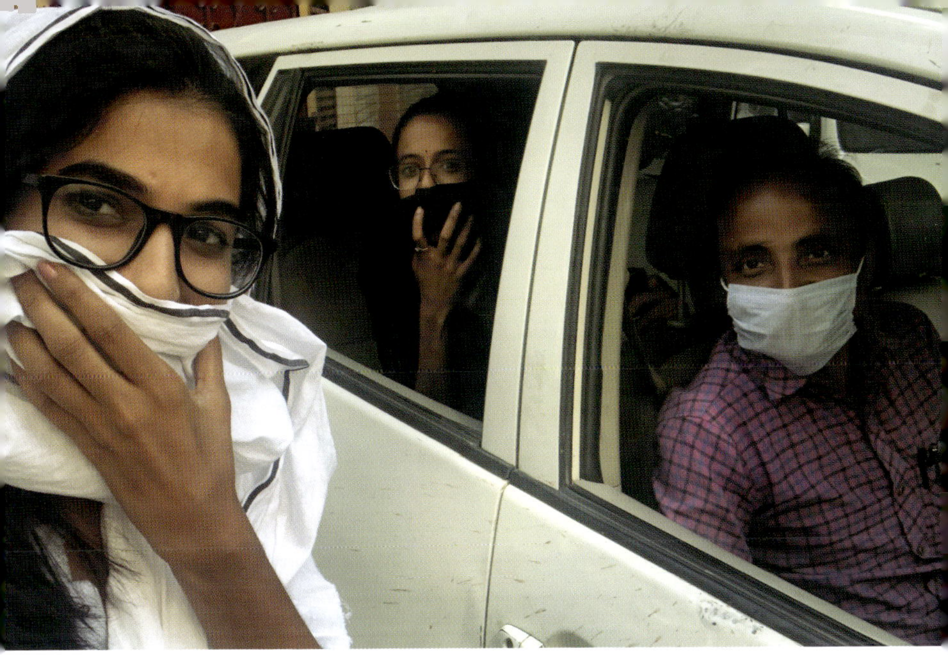

A selfie taken before Manish, Bismee and I went our separate ways in Delhi after the assignment ended

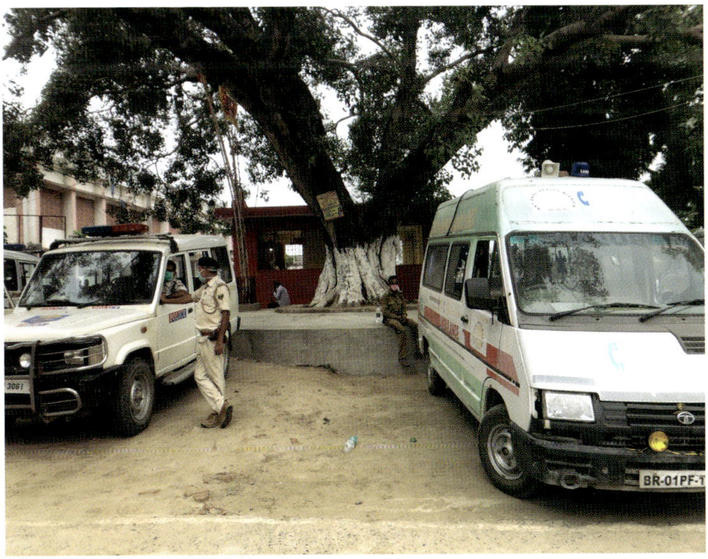

A police escort accompanied an ambulance that ferried the bodies of migrants killed in an accident on their final journey home—from Naugachia in Bhagalpur to Bettiah and Motihari districts.

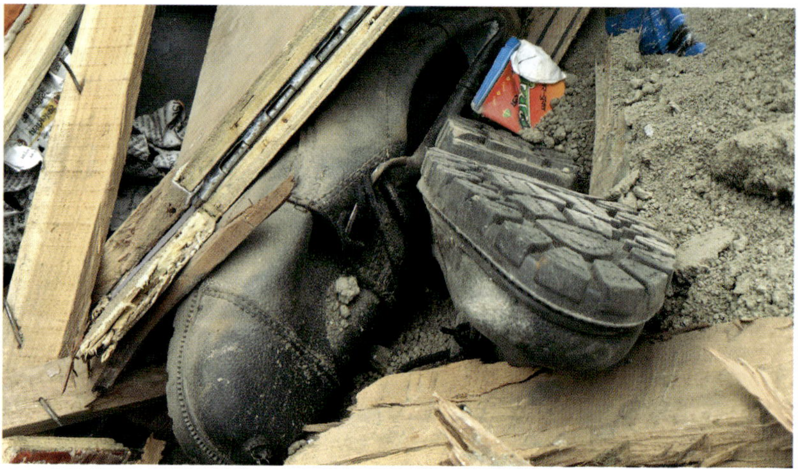

At the accident site in Naugachia, torn shoes, ripped clothes, and remnants of food lay scattered along National Highway 31. The migrants were still eight hours away from home when they were brutally killed in the crash.

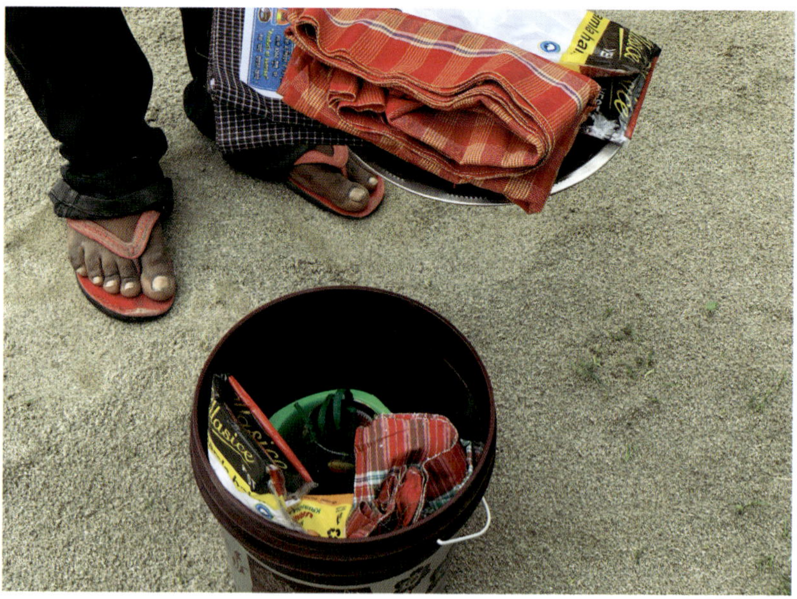

A migrant shows his dignity kit, provided by the Nitish Kumar government to those isolated in quarantine centres. The kit included sixteen items—combs, soaps, buckets, mosquito nets, bedsheets, etc.

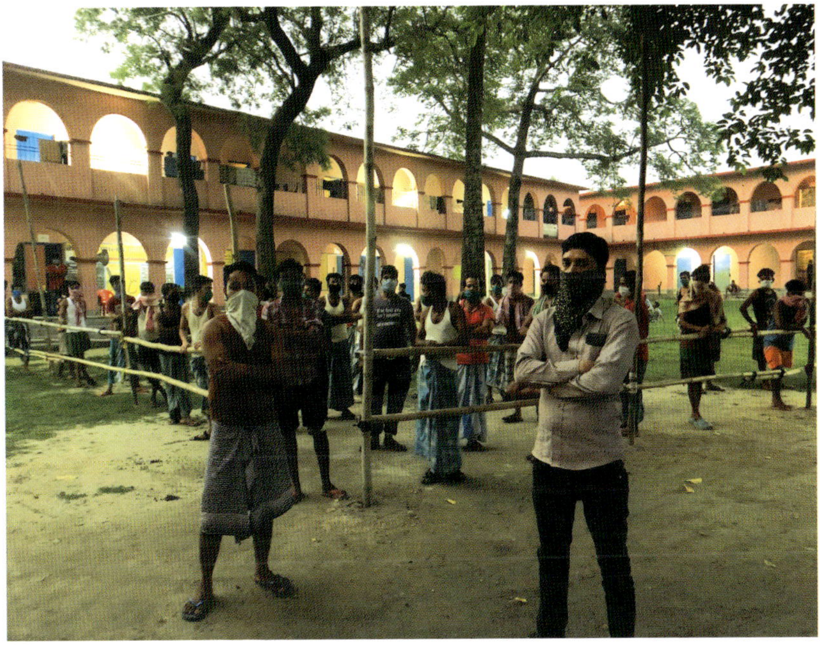

This school-turned-quarantine centre in the Barsoi block of Katihar district was barricaded with bamboo poles to enforce isolation and social distancing. But with hundreds of migrants packed into just four-five rooms, distancing was impossible.

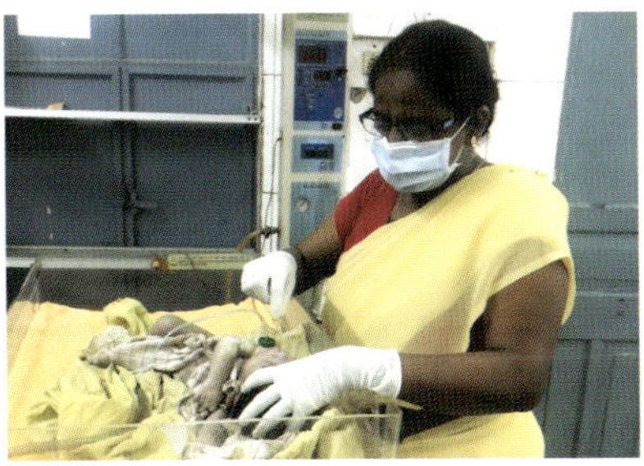

Rekha Devi and Sandeep Yadav's fifth child— a girl—was born at the district hospital in Gopalganj. A nurse was cleaning the newborn. The nurses were hesitant for fear of COVID until the collector intervened, and two lives were saved.

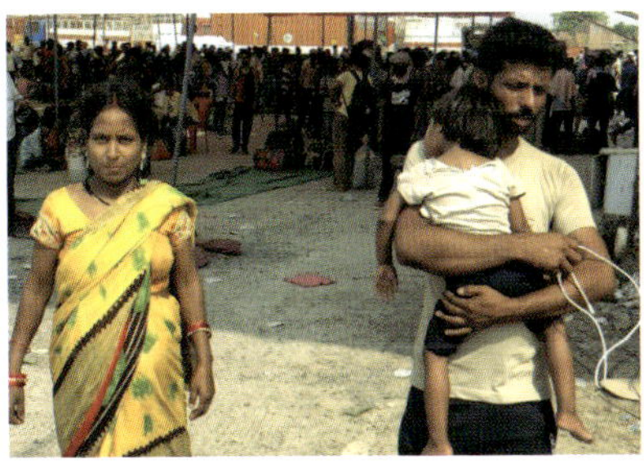

Rekha had travelled nearly 900 kilometres from Noida, while nine months pregnant, at the peak of the migrant exodus. We met her amidst the sea of exhausted migrants at a transit centre on the Gopalganj border, just hours before she gave birth.

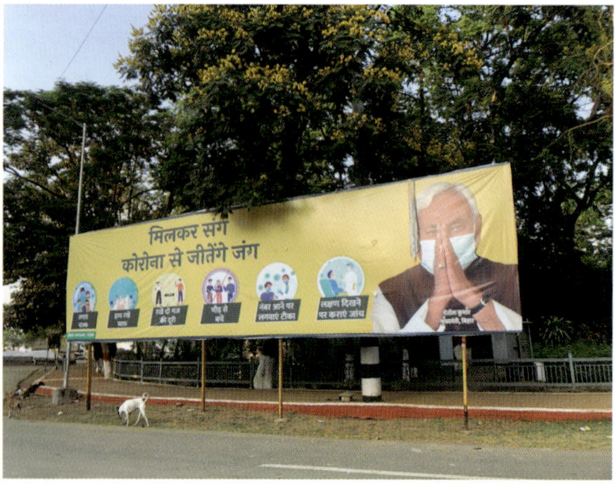

A hoarding in Patna shows Chief Minister Nitish Kumar with folded hands and a masked face, assuring: 'Together, we will defeat the virus.'

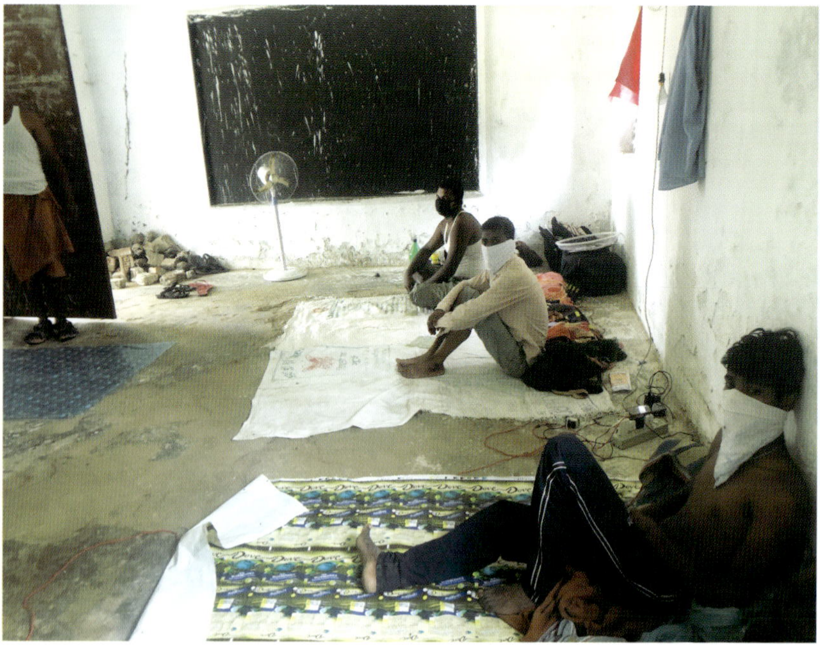

A quarantine centre in Manihari block of Katihar district in Seemanchal Bihar, where returned migrants completed a mandatory isolation phase before being allowed back into their village community.

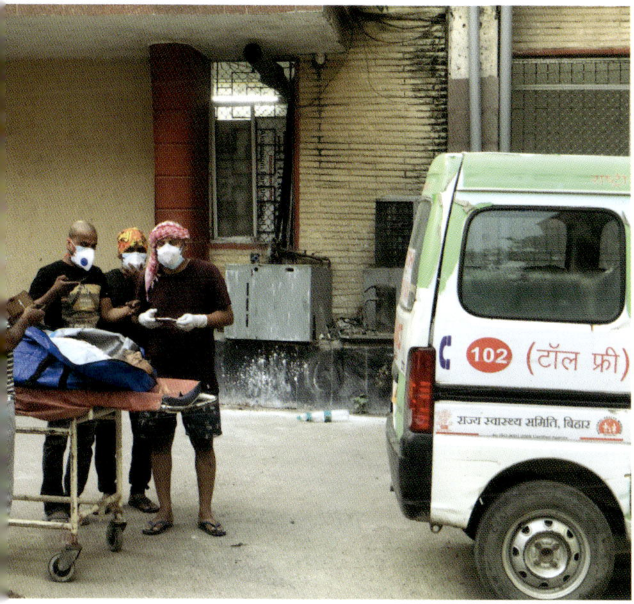

The body of 71-year-old Bhagwat Rai lay surrounded by his four sons. They demanded that it be unwrapped to make sure his kidneys and eyes had not been stolen. The sons took multiple photos of their deceased father. Just days earlier, Bhagwat Rai's wife, Lakhi Devi, had lost her life to COVID-19.

In the corridors of Patna's NMCH, a staffer was cleaning as Amitesh (seen wearing a helmet) ran from pillar to post, trying to secure a ventilator for his 56-year-old mother, Sheela Kumari.

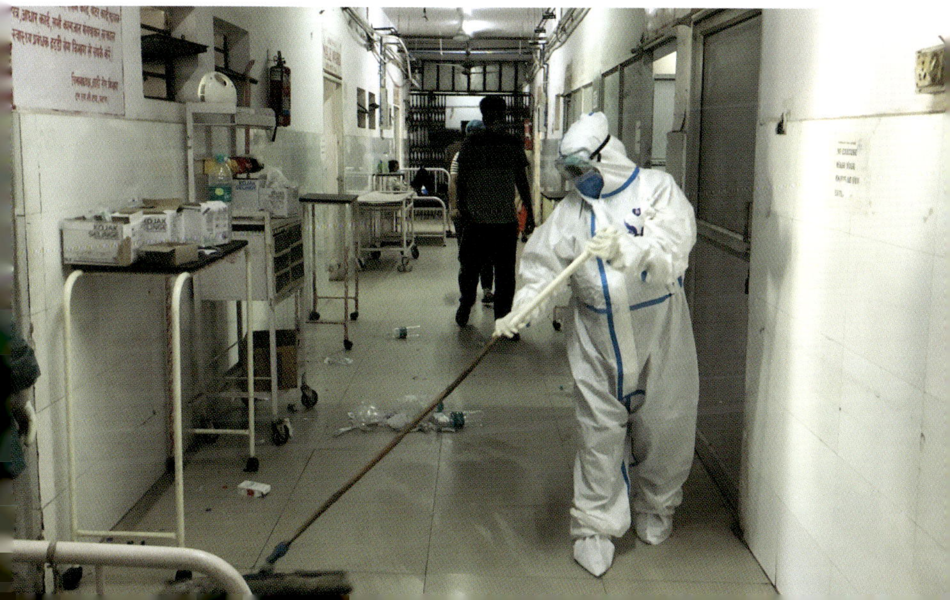

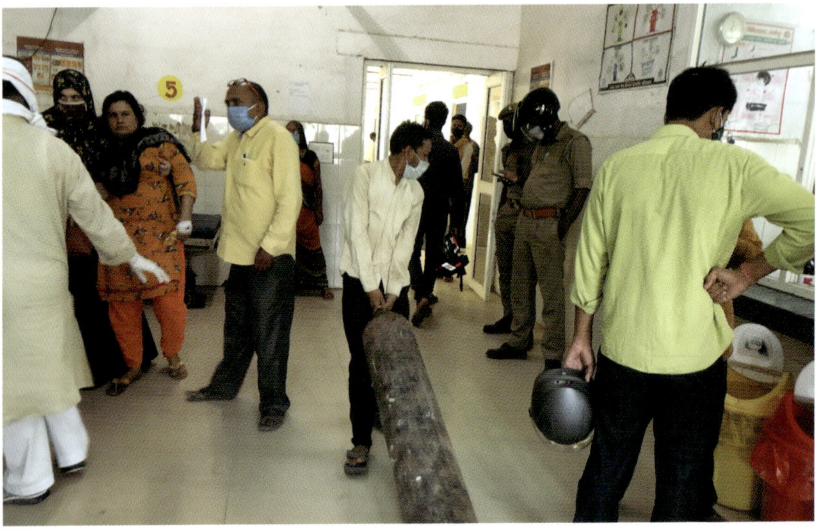

In the general ward of the district hospital in Ghazipur, a man drags an oxygen cylinder through the crowd, while others stand wearing helmets, gamchhas and cloth masks as makeshift shields. The second COVID wave was at its peak at this moment.

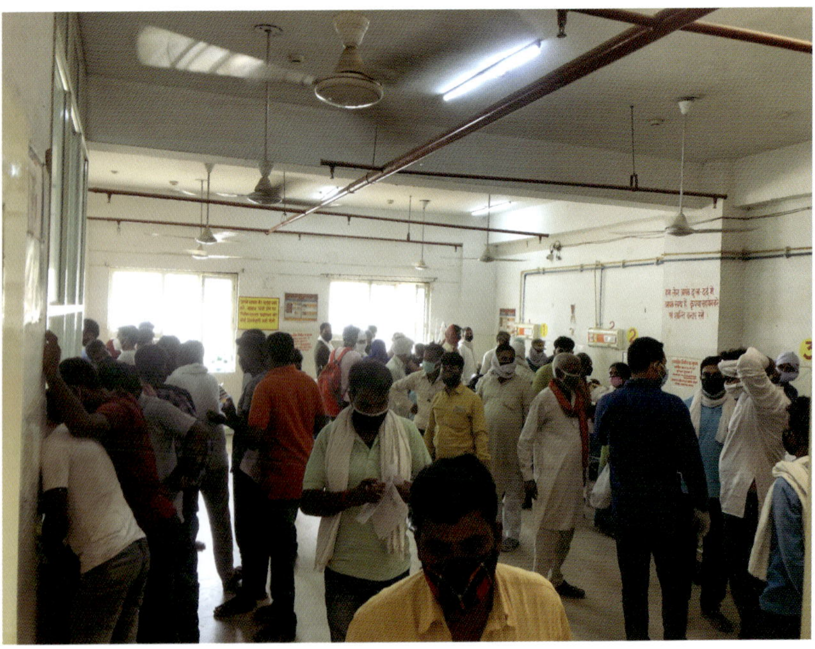

The general ward at the district hospital in Ghazipur, Uttar Pradesh, overflowing with patients and harried attendants.